HOLISTIC HEALTH

HOLISTIC
HEALTH

by Dr. Robert E. Duke

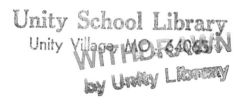
New Horizon Press
Far Hills, New Jersey

The opinions in this book are exclusively those of the author, and do not necessarily reflect the opinions of the publisher.

Manufactured in the United States of America   7-86

Library of Congress Cataloging in Publication Data
Duke, Robert E.
   Holistic Health
Includes index.
1. Health. 2. Holistic medicine. 3. Exercise.
4. Mind and body. I. Title
RA776.5.D85   1985   613 8515376

ISBN 0-88282-011-7

HOLISTIC HEALTH

Everyone should be his own physician. We ought to assist, not force nature. What medicine can procure digestion? Excercise. What will recruit strength? Sleep. What will alleviate incurable evils? Patience.

—Voltaire

TABLE OF CONTENTS

REMARKS

H.R.H. Charles, The Prince of Wales, reasserts the historical concept of healing the whole human being when he states:

"By concentrating on smaller and smaller fragments of the body modern medicine perhaps loses sight of the patient as a whole human being, and by reducing health to mechanical functioning it is no longer able to deal with the phenomenon of healing. And here I come back to my original point. The term "healer" is viewed with suspicion and the concepts of health and healing are probably not generally discussed enough in medical schools. But to reincorporate the notion of healing into the practice of medicine does not necessarily mean that medical science will have to be less scientific. Through the centuries healing has been practised by folk-healers who are guided by traditional wisdom that sees illness as a disorder of the whole person, involving not only the patient's body, but his mind, his self-image, his dependence on the physical and social environment, as well as his relation to the cosmos. Paracelsus constantly repeated the old adage that "Nature heals, the doctor nurses"—and it is well to remember that these sort of healers still treat the majority of patients throughout the world. Some of them, in the form of black Christian bishops in Africa, are subjected to the most appalling kind of mis-informed abuse and censure, which so characterized the world elements of missionary activity amongst populations whose childlike acceptance of the symbols of life and of Nature is one of their most endearing and vital qualities.

I would suggest that the whole imposing edifice of modern medicine for all its breath-taking success is, like the celebrated Tower of Pisa, slightly off balance. No-one of course could be stupid enough to deny the enormous benefits which the advances of medical science in this century have conferred upon us all. To take only one example—penicillin administered in a case of infective heart disease leads to survival in an illness otherwise uniformly fatal. Anyone who has had this kind of experience is likely to be a powerful supporter of modern methods in medicine, but nevertheless the fact remains that contemporary medicine as a whole tends to be fascinated by the objective, statistical, computerized approach to the healing of the sick. If disease is regarded as an objective problem isolated from all personal factors, then surgery plus more and more powerful drugs must be the answer. Already the cost of drugs supplied to patients by the N.H.S. alone is well over £2000 million a year. It is frightening how dependent upon drugs we are all becoming and how easy it is for doctors to prescribe them as the universal panacea for our ills. Wonderful as many of them are it should still be more widely stressed by doctors that the health of human beings is so often determined by their behaviour, their food and the nature of their environment."

ACKNOWLEDGMENTS

The author would like to acknowledge the work of Dr. George H. Taylor and Dr. Charles Fayette Taylor who studied the work of Professor Peter Henry Ling of Sweden. It was Professor Ling who developed the gymnastic movement that restored the health, strength and beauty of many Swedish people. Professor Ling was born at Smaland in 1766. This is also the birth place of my own great-grandfather.

Professor Ling developed and taught his curative movements in Stockholm, where he founded the Central Institute, an academy devoted to this work. His public support increased and he was eventually knighted by his sovereign.

The doctors Taylor studied Professor Ling's achievements and published them in the United States. Much of my research is based on Professor Ling's original achievements as told by the two doctors. Innovative theories based on their findings have given new support to our current renewal of interest in holistic healing.

INTRODUCTION

As Albert Schweitzer the noted humanitarian and healer once explained, the true doctor simply awakens "the physician within" to achieve ultimate health for the patient's mind and body. The principles of holistic health which this book explores illustrate how this self-restorative process can be accomplished. Some of the measures it advocates are: organic foods to replace chemically infested diets, natural herbs instead of drug therapy, yoga, self-hypnosis, and a system of physical therapy by movements—to slim the body, cure chronic diseases, and open up new frontiers of well-being. Real healing and consummate health, however, entail not only these curative therapies, but also a radical change in philosophical values and beliefs.

Holistic health as a way of life prescribes that we discard the disunified view that humanity is separate from nature and that we see all living things as a part of the totality of life. In this way, enlightened self-interest is consistent with greater well-being and we can discover the wisdom of wholeness. This wisdom has been practiced by the Chinese, Japanese, Hebrews, Indians, Hawaiians, Egyptians, and early Greek philosophers. To practice the principles of holistic health we must return to the guidance of such ancient wisdom. But such practice also demands the judicious use of the best of modern Western therapy combined with the best of ancient health practices from East and West—old and new.

Looking at revolutionary health practices around the world, those which astound us most are often examples of the ancient wisdom of wholeness. For instance:

In France, an obstetrician eliminates the pain of childbirth through hypnosis;

In China, an acupuncturist extracts a tooth without discomfort by placing several needles at strategic pressure points;

In India, a man lies for three days upon a bed of nails;

In Ireland, a healer causes a blind man to see;

In New York, a medium locates a dead body in Central Park.

To ponder about the wonders of such feats is to begin to contemplate the challenge of wholeness proposed by holistic wisdom.

Whether the problem is understanding the reasons for overweight, chronic disease, mental suffering, or so-called "miracles," neither the affliction nor the cure is rendered in isolation. Human beings are composed of body, mind, and spirit. The needs of these three components must be considered and balanced, as must the relationships of all things to each other.

No one can totally extricate him or herself from the detrimental external environment of modern society: pollution, noise, emotional stress, acid rain. The negative effects resulting from these influences on our bodies cannot be ignored. However, if one accepts the holistic principles of health and disease, and with courage and conviction cultivates the wisdom of the body—the connection between body sensitivity and mind awareness—which has been almost lost to most of modern civilization, then the restorative process leading to well-being can begin.

Understanding the intricate interrelationships of nature will teach that cures cannot be broken up and fragmented. A person who exercises frequently but eats a garbage diet of chemically infested foods will not function well for very long. It is not only our physical lifestyles, but our mental lifestyles as well that need revitalization. Dieting for one week will not help chronic overweight. Exercising for short periods will not firm flabby muscles. Nor will infrequent periods of rest and meditation end susceptibility to stress.

Everyday life is where permanent changes must be effected and a balance maintained. By treating the mind and body as a whole and providing remedies that encompass the entire lifestyle of an individual, by effecting changes in one's dietary and emotional environments, chronic degenerative and psychosomatic disorders can be overcome and the natural health processes within that person will function effectively to prevent disease, promote health, and combat the pressures of daily life in a complex society.

Through the techniques of holistic health, every individual can learn to be a self-healer and influence the mind—ultimately directly affecting the body. Thus, holistic healing will provide the ultimate therapy for mind, body, and spirit. By practicing its rules, we can open up new frontiers of well-being and live longer, more fulfilling lives. Do it for your health's sake!

1   Principles of Holistic Therapy

"Judy was a full term, seemingly healthy baby. We brought her home weighing seven pounds and thriving but for the next six months she screamed day and night with colic. We went to three pediatricians, but none of them could find a physical cause. Finally, one sent us to an allergist. Her allergies turned out to be non-specific. She continued to look bloated at times, have sleepless periods and was constantly irritable."

Toby spent several days every few weeks riddled by the severe pain of migraines. Her successive doctors had prescribed everything from codeine to Demerol, but as she put it, "my headaches still cripple me. I've tried every kind of specialist and every kind of pill. Nothing works. Do I have to continue to suffer? The last doctor told me to try psychoanalysis. Am I crazy?"

Charley was the head of sales for a prominent insurance firm. He traveled constantly, entertained lavishly, consumed alcohol with hectic speed in order to slow down in the evening, and by his bedside kept a giant bottle of antacid pills which he chewed on throughout the night whenever the stomach distress from the ulcer he had developed awoke him.

Apathetic and despondent, Jenna, a nineteen year old former college student had already been hospitalized twice for suicide attempts. She ate little and her physical appearance had begun to take on anorexic qualities. Moreover, she had stopped going out except when absolutely necessary. "I'm hopeless," she kept murmuring again and again.

All of these illnesses have many causes. No one factor alone causes them nor can one magic pill cure them. The remedy for many of the ills I have been describing is neither to consume enormous amounts of chemicals ranging from stomach and headache relievers to anti-depressents and amphetamines nor to seek out a super-surgeon or internist, but to reassess our current health-care practices and to recognize that the huge amount of money we spend treating chronic illnesses and prevent-able diseases is often not achieving our aim—good health.

Good health and health treatment are not the same. Personal, environmental and spiritual factors affect each human being's optimal well-being. Only through the harmonious functioning of mind and body can one be sensitive to the inner wisdom which lies within every one of us. This intuitive knowledge has great self-healing power. It has been expressed by Nobel prize winner

Albert Saint Georgio as "the drive in living matter to perfect itself."

When Judy, the baby in our example, was fed a natural diet, her environment cleansed of its major toxins, and physical movement therapy initiated, she became the beautiful child it was her potential to be.

Yoga, diet and hypnosis largely rid Toby of the energy-depleting headaches from which she had suffered for so long. Moreover, the relaxation techniques she learned brought her closer to the inner peace and fulfillment for which she yearned.

Charley came to realize that his high-pressure life which had brought him the benefits of success had also brought him the pain of a serious physical condition. For Charley, the choice seemed difficult but an episode of internal bleeding and subsequent hospitalization caused him to see the need for changing his lifestyle.

The hopelessness Jenna felt was caused primarily, because she had given up on herself. She was involved with no one and her feelings of loneliness were so intense that she was subconsciously starving herself to death in order to escape. The prescribed anti-depressant intensified her physical affliction while lowering her anxiety and awareness. Meditative and self-hypnotic techniques, diet and exercise helped Jenna tap her own healing resources.

All of these people sought holistic healing, because

they had tried endless doctors, medications and conventional treatments without attaining health. As a last alternative, having come to distrust the tools of technological medicine, harmful and habit-forming drugs, excessive surgery and x-rays, they began to explore the possibilities of a holistic, humane and natural approach to healing. A whole new world of physical and spiritual well-being opened to them; once they were willing to call upon nature—her remedies, her antidotes, her prescriptions—and to use these as adjuncts to their own natural abilities to heal themselves. Flowing with the currents of life, each finally learned to achieve a balance of body-mind-spirit and to become a vitally alive whole person. In truth, they healed themselves.

The responsibility for health, and happiness falls upon the shoulders of everybody. Nature has endowed human beings with the means for adapting themselves to their environment and maintaining their health systems in perfect order. They have been provided with the intelligence that is often needed to reverse and control chance and accidents.

Human beings have always wanted to be as complete, attractive, vigorous, and healthy as they can. The desire to be an ideal person has existed throughout all ages. This desire is rooted in our subconscious mind and our physiology.

Holistic therapy may be the best way to give direction to these desires. The principle is a hygienic and remedial art based on the natural harmonious operations of the body and mind. Through such training, mind and body become more perfect.

The value of Holistic therapy has never been denied but it has been abandoned for the alternative of drug therapy; as a result the pharmaceutical industry in America has flourished. More and more, chemistry is furnishing medical practice with a means of toying with the hopes and fears of the suffering public's credulity.

The principles of Holistic therapy described in this book are inimical to the interests of medical practice. They are based upon common sense and truth, and to a large extent will enable people to dispense with drug-style medication and sedentary lifestyles.

It must be conceded that medical science doesn't answer many of the requirements of our civilization; its scope is too narrow. It does not even attempt to address our complex problems properly, because its chief aim is not to keep us well, but to find a mighty cure-all. And through such practices the limited resources of many individuals are exhausted.

Current medical practice depends upon the belief that there really is a connection between drugs and certain curative results. It seems obvious that the implied promise of the medical profession to cure through drugs, lessens the fear of pain, which is the penalty men pay for their own physiological mis-treatment.

We need to look more closely at the principles involved in drug-practice. Does an expected drug-cure discourage inquiry into the actual physiological factors of an illness? Does it offer an indulgence for physiological neglect? Does the promise of drug-cure annihilate the fear of illness? If not, to what else do we attribute the general ignorance and indifference to physical and mental culture which modern medicine often promotes.

Suppose there were no drug treatments for physiological neglect and that suffering and diminished power were its direct and inevitable consequence. Would this stimulate inquiry and lead us to practice holistic therapy? I think so, because self-preservation and self-interest would leave us no alternative.

The need for special physical and mental hygiene and culture to help the recovering invalids, the elderly, the weak, those individuals whose jobs require too little or improper exercise, and the youth of both sexes must be manifest to all. The importance of holistic therapy as a curative resource is second to none.

One purpose of this book is to promote a part of this theory that is based upon movement in the human body. These movements, practiced long ago in Eastern cultures, have been called "movements" and they will work wonders for just about everybody. The various applications of the movements contained herein provide individuals from every walk of life with a powerful supplementary tool for a healthy life.

Exercise has an incontrovertible remedial effect, and therefore has an integral role in the prevention and treatment of disease. The use of the exercise-cure has been known and practiced—to a limited extent—throughout the ages and in many cultures. It is not now nor ever has been offered as a universal panacea. It is a valuable contribution that embraces every avenue through which the health of the body is influenced, by either external or internal causes.

Medical practice tends to limit treatment to the use of drugs but these constitute only one class of agents involved in good health. Other contributing agents are those that relate to man as an animal—such as heat, cold, food, drink, labor, recreation, rest—and all the inter-relationships of these with the functions of the body.

The holistic cure system regards man as both a physical and spiritual being, recognizing all the influences on his life affected by mental and physical causes; the power of mind over bodily functions. The fact that these influences directly modify and control health is unquestionable. This control can be used as a remedial means for physical well-being and mental powers can exercise control over the nervous states and over the body functions that effect health. In this book I will show how the co-operating mental and physical effects may be further developed into a healing system called holistic therapy.

I will explore two major therapies: mental exercises and physiological exercises. Either can be considered a means of encouraging the natural tendencies of the system to react more potently and effectively and thus produce excellent health. Together, they enable the system to develop and maintain its vital energy-producing healing forces because they employ them naturally.

2   Holistic Body Power

We must know something about the nature, origin and relationships of the powers of the body if we are to direct them toward good health. The kind of health we possess is determined by the kinds of actions that are going on in our physical being; the powers of the body depend upon these actions. In other words, bodily health is referable to conditions, or good or ill feelings, which we superficially regard as constituting well-being. Hence, medical control of health essentially consists in control of these elementary actions. Medical practice that does not recognize the changes induced on these primary actions as the basis and explanation of power is empirical and appeals chiefly to the sensations, which are not worthy of reliance. When a sick person is made comfortable by means of a drug, he is satisfied that its effects are good and is disinclined to investigate further. Often what this patient has received has only placebo value, he or she is not made healthy again.

To establish and maintain two great forces is the main objective of all operations in the human system. These are the mechanical and nervous forces. All the bodily functions and actions are subservient to these chief purposes.

The mechanical forces include the great mass of the flesh of the body covering the skeleton, while the nervous forces are by their filaments, extensively and minutely distributed to the muscles and all other parts of the body, as well as existing in distinct local masses in the head and central portions of the body. The nervous forces are of several distinct classes, each sustaining peculiar relationships to the organism, but all associated into one grand unit. These classes are: the sensorial and intellectual, relating to the mind; the reflex, connecting the mind and senses with the muscles, the medium of mechanical power; and the organic, relating to the various agencies concerned with growth.

These powerful instruments create the individuality and distinctive character of the man, the grade and quality of his being. It is through these that he impresses surrounding things, acts upon them in a thousand ways, and modifies their relationships to assist his purposes and desires. It is through the use of these agents that he attempts to understand the designs of nature and God, discovering the laws that explain his surroundings things and his own spiritual nature. The possession of these powers fulfills his utmost desires. These powers are capable of progressive and almost limitless expansion, but they *may* act inharmoniously, feebly, painfully, or antagonistically.

The latter condition constitutes disease. We must go to the source of these disease manifestations if we are to correct or improve them.

To improve these capabilities and to train them in their proper uses is to put an individual in possession of his healing powers. Ill health is evidence of loss of such control; mostly medical efforts are merely endeavors to temporarily restore this control.

In order to acquire balance and perfection in the powers of the mind, the necessity of training the mind through exercise has been acknowledged by all societies, from the most rudimentary to the most civilized.

The vital acts through which animal power is manifested may be included under the general term *nutrition*. The term covers the total process whereby the integrity of the organism is preserved. It consists of many distinct actions, whether chemically or physiologically considered. These actions are resolvable into two general classes which, in good health, are nicely balanced. These classes are named construction and destruction of organic forms.

In effecting these functional acts two distinct classes of materials are employed in the body, both of which are conveyed to the scene of vital activity by the blood. These are food and oxygen—one entering the blood through the stomach, by means of digestion, the other through the lungs, by respiration.

The general purpose of these materials is to maintain the actions that produce the two classes of effects under consideration: the food to build up, and the oxygen to change, by its chemical power, the composition of organic bodies, and to reduce them to the state in which they exit from the body.

Since the chief intention of the processes within the

body is either to build up or to demolish, it follows that all the influences brought into action with the organism must tend to promote one or the other of these results. Such is the normal intention of food and oxygen, both of which are received into the system in about equal quantities. The product of the digestion of food is employed in the organizing processes, while the oxygen aids in dissolving these organized molecules into a soluble or volatile form, thereby facilitating their exit from the system.

When the influences exerted upon the physiological processes are such as to promote equally and properly these actions of waste and renewal, health is the natural consequence. The theory and practice of the principles concerned in the maintenance of good health are incorporated in the term, hygiene.

Holistic Hygiene is understood to be the intelligent application of certain principles and agents for the restoration of lost or impaired health. The employment of physical-culture movements is a powerful means of directing or enforcing nutrition. Physical movements are devices for aiding the organism in its efforts to derive sustenance from suitable materials, and for assisting the exit of waste matters; thus constituting a special application of hygiene. Hygiene, in general, embraces the means that are influential in controlling the waste and renewal of the body.

All substances incapable of supporting the growth of the vital parts will modify and generally accelerate the wasting processes of the body.

All substances which are incapable of supporting the

growth of the vital parts, and this includes drugs, will modify and generally accelerate the wasting processes of the body. When a living molecule is contacted by a drug which has been introduced into the system, the natural affinity of the molecule for oxygen is increased, or it is impressed by the chemical or mechanical effects of the foreign substance. The symptoms are the result of the unusual waste and the consequent rapid evolution of the intermediate forms of wasting matter. This makes the ejection of these matters more difficult—distending the capillaries of the affected part and resulting in discomfort and pain.

Drugs are often classified as to how they effect certain pathological conditions. They may be considered to be favoring the chemical changes in the body—sometimes accelerating, sometimes impeding the manifestation of power, but never promoting the production of that power, by contributing to the primary organizing processes.

Good health depends upon positive changes occurring in the human being which improve the regular condition. The incentives for the changes can be physiological or psychological in nature or a composite of both.

3   Holistic Hygiene

By holistic hygiene we mean rules and regulations which we apply to our conduct and mode of living. Among the areas covered are food, drink, air temperature, light, exercise, and mental attitudes.

A substance is a food if, when introduced into the stomach, it is capable of sustaining the vital actions of the system. Its efficiency in this role depends on such factors as quantity, quality, method of preparation, times of eating, etc.

Food which serves nutritive purposes does so through oxygen; consequently the quantity of food to be used is limited by respiration and the factors effecting it. We are unconscious of the rate of the oxidizing process going on within us so we are guided in our food intake almost entirely by our sensations. The necessities of the system are absolute but the sensations are subject to variations from many different and changing causes. Therefore, deciding the proper amount of food to be eaten at a given time is difficult, especially for those whose gastric systems are deranged.

Errors in quantity are liable to occur for the following reasons:

1. In disease the amount of oxidized products eliminated from the system is greatly reduced. Thus the amount of food consumed should be reduced accordingly. In acute disease the results are a lessened affinity of blood for oxygen are rendered conspicious in the character of the urine, the fur of the tongue, and quickened pulse and respiration—which is an attempt to compensate for this lessened affinity. In either case no restoration is possible while there continues to be an excess of food over respiration.

2. Bodily inactivity reduces the need of the system for food, and the ill effect of consuming the same amount of food as when actively employed soon becomes apparent in lessened health.

3. Elevated temperature necessarily diminishes the amount of carbonic acid and water produced in the system. Consequently the amount of food required is less than is demanded at low temperatures.

4. Confinement in close rooms, out of the reach of fresh air, diminishes the amount of oxygen taken into the system both by skin and lungs.

5. Anything taken into the stomach that unduly stimulates it, such as spices, sweets, condiments, and prescribed drugs, perverts and blunts the sensibility of the organ, and inclines it to solicit an undue quantity of food.

That portion of alimentary material taken into the system over and above what it needs, must be regarded as foreign matter over which the organism can exercise, at best, an imperfect control.

Food consists of materials capable of being organized or transformed into the vital structure and of materials which are only oxidized in the body and reduced to a form easy of elimination. The former class contains nitrogen, the latter does not. The nitrogenized class is of uniform composition, represented by albumen and by its modifications, fibrin, gluten, casein, etc. No other substances containing nitrogen are capable of being transformed into the instruments of life. The non-nitrogenized class is represented by starch, sugar, vegetable acids, etc.

The errors common in the quality of food are chiefly:

1. The distinction between proper food and other matters destined to oxidation in the system is frequently lost sight of. In this way such substances as alcohol and its various mixtures have come to be considered as food.

2. A good proportion of the saline constituents of food essential to nutrition is lost in the mechanical separation effected by the milling of grain.

3. The habitual use of food dissolved in water is fruitless. The system provides secretions in proportion to its needs for nourishment. If the food is already dissolved, or soluble in water, it may pass into circulation even though it is injurious to the system.

4. The supposition that adding spices to food is essential or useful is very common—and erroneous. Spices only detract from the nutritive value of food and do harm by forcing the system to labor in their elimination.

5. There is a disproportion in the nutritive elements taken into the system. Indulgence in sweets overloads

the blood with hydrocarbons and diminishes the relative proportion of the nitrogenized and organizable constitutents of food.

The objective of cooking should not be to change the intrinsic chemical qualities of food. It does not add to, and may even detract from, the nutritive qualities in most cases although there are a few instances where noxious qualities of plants are eliminated by cooking.

Cooking should be used to increase the digestibility of food. It renders the nutritive properties promptly available to the digestive organs with the aid of heat and moisture which softens fibers, opens starch granules, softens woody fibers, and reduces the mechanical labor of the digestive organs to the lowest practical point.

The mistakes most commonly used in cooking involve the use of unnecessarily high temperatures which injure food's nutritive properties (bread, for instance, is toasted and the juices of meats are burned to gratify an acquired taste); sugar, oily matters, alkalies, etc., are commonly added to food, utterly disregarding the needs of the system; and food is rendered so porous and soft that it is swallowed without chewing, depriving it of the saliva needed for its proper digestion.

The proper times for eating are hard to pin down. People who work are apt to have long intervals between meals; if the intervals are not too extended, however, this may even be beneficial.

In sedentary life, especially for those who are ill, there is often a preoccupation with food and a temptation to eat more frequently.

In the case of a stomach ailment, the demand on the

digestive organs for nutritive material lessens and the digestive process is conducted with less energy. Thus, the need for food is experienced less frequently and it would be a hazard to the health to eat as much as is required when not ailing. A good rule to observe is to eat nothing while any of the preceding meal remains in the stomach. The residual food acts as a ferment, hindering the succeeding digestive effort. It may be necessary in some cases to extend the time between meals to effect a purification of the solvent fluids.

In a state of health the digestive process proceeds in stages and requires time. Introduction of food or drink at the wrong time tends to arrest the process and render it ineffective.

Water is the only substance which can be considered a wholesome beverage. All artificial drinks consist of various mixtures, infusions, or solutions of other matters—either solid or liquid—with water. So, tea, coffee and alcohol are beverages due only to the water they contain. To consider the physiological relations of these drinks is to investigate the effect of their chemicals upon the vital bodily structures. They have been shown to contribute, not to nutrition, but to irritation, stimulation, and destruction of organized substances. Their use, in any form, is incompatible with remedial treatment.

Milk is frequently drunk by adults as well as by children. It consists of about eighty percent water holding about twenty percent solid matter in solution. The largest portion of the solid matter immediately precipitates upon reaching the stomach. Milk can clog the system by loading it with too much nutritive matter. This is incompatible with the systems of some people.

There is natural salt in the blood system so that the human body does not need constant replenishment of its salt supply. The salt retained by the blood serves its purposes over and over again. Any salt appearing in the excretions is in excess of the system's needs and if this condiment is consumed in large quantities, salt can be detrimental and overwork the kidneys. Some physiologists regard salt as a poison and they cite cases of edema and hypertension to support their belief.

Recent surveys show that 15 percent of all adults have some degree of hypertension and would benefit from reduced sodium intake. The excessive use of saline substances is the gravest error in modern dietetics.

Vegetarian diets are becoming increasingly popular as the belief spreads that a properly planned vegetarian diet can provide all the essential nutrients. It appears true that quasi-vegetarians (those who eat fish) are less likely to be afflicted with chronic crippling diseases. Some claim their diet eliminates arthritis, depression and even vaginal infections.

There are definitive studies that suggest benefits in a reduction of fat-containing animal foods and an increase in the consumption of vegetables and whole grains in lowering the level of blood fats, cholesterol and triglycerides. High levels of blood fats are associated with an increased risk of heart disease.

Lacto-ovo vegetarians, those who eat eggs and dairy products (which contain cholesterol-raising saturated fats), have higher blood fat levels than do strict vegetarians.

A Boston study* revealed that when eight ounces of meat were added to the daily diet of strict vegetarians for four weeks, blood-cholesterol levels rose by 19 percent, even though the volunteers gained no weight.

It appears that while eliminating meat from the diet is likely to reduce the fats and cholesterol, substituting large amounts of high-fat dairy products and eggs can negate such benefits. In order to benefit from vegetarianism, the use of such foods as hard cheese, cream cheese, ice cream and eggs should be moderate or eliminated completely.

High blood pressure tends to occur more often among meat eaters than among vegetarians. In his book, *The Vegetarian Alternative*, published by Rodale Press in 1980, Vick Sussman cites a recent study conducted in Israel which showed that of 200 people, only 2 percent of the vegetarians had high blood pressure compared to 26 percent of nonvegetarians of the same age and circumstances. A similar study conducted in Finland also reported a significant decline in blood pressure when the participants switched to low-fat diets. Many other studies give the same warnings.

Cancer of the breast, colon and prostate are more common worldwide among the people who eat a high-fat, high-meat, low-fiber diet. In the United States, the Seventh Day Adventists who follow vegetarian diets are only half as likely as the average American to develop

*Quincy Patriot Ledger. Quincy, Mass. February 1, 1984

cancer of the colon or rectum. They also have a lower rate of cancer of the breast, ovary, prostate and pancreas.

On the average, people who follow vegetarian diets are leaner than meat eaters and many people who switch to a vegetarian diet lose weight. Only 15 percent of vegetarian Seventh Day Adventists are overweight, as compared to 30 percent to 40 percent of meat-eating people. In addition to a lower fat intake, vegetarians eat more low-calorie vegetables and dietary fiber which tends to fill them up before they have consumed too many calories.

There is much good that can be said for a vegetarian's diet. Nowadays, some women even have polluting chemicals in their breast milk; it seems that the chemicals enter the human body as a contaminant of animal fat and are stored in the human body. The cancer-initiating factors called mutagens that are produced when meat is broiled or fried are lower in a vegetarian diet. Also, since vegetarians tend to eat less protein and phosphorous than meat-eaters, their calcium requirements tend to be lower and thereby reduce the risk of osteoporosis (loss of calcium from the bones).

Here are some common folk remedies, utilizing food sources, which will restore and improve your health.

Honey. This is both a basic food and a food supplement. It has already been digested by bees and perhaps this is why it is so quickly absorbed into the human gastrointestinal tract. It has a mild laxative effect and is a sedative for those in need of a sound sleep. Expectant mothers who ingest one or two tablespoons of honey with their meals can expect to help their infant develop a better nervous system. Honey has also been used to help alcoholics overcome their addiction. Modern foods, because of the way they are over-processed, are robbed of their natural mineral contents. It seems that some of those minerals, which alcoholics need, can be found in honey. When this need is satisfied the alcoholic is more likely to overcome his addiction. Honey contains iron, copper, manganese, silica, chlorine, calcium, potassium, sodium, phosphorus, aluminum and manganese.

Honey is also an important source of vitamins; in fact, honey contains all the vitamins that are necessary for good health.

Honey has also been effective in relieving hay fever. If possible, the honey should be obtained directly from the beekeeper together with the honey comb. It is suggested that the hay fever sufferer chew the honey comb along with the honey and swallow the substance. If this is difficult then the wax can be spit out after it has been chewed very throughly. The author of this book was bothered by this affliction and healed in this way. An individual suffering from annual attacks of great severity should start this program several months before the hay fever season begins and continue with it until the season is over.

Kelp. Ocean kelp contains many of the minerals needed by the human body, in a compatible organic form. Sea plants may be the richest source of the vital substances required for health. There are some maritime people who use the resources of the sea and consume large quantities of kelp. The Japanese and the Irish consume comparatively large quantities of edible seaweeds and, as a result, don't suffer the associated diet deficiency diseases. The average Japanese eats about ten grains of dried kelp every day.

Kelp has also been used successfully to treat heart pain. The quantity suggested is one five-grain tablet at each meal. The kelp and the seaweed called *dulce* is available in selected grocery and health food stores.

Iodine. One important mineral found in kelp is iodine which contributes to the proper functioning of the thyroid gland. Dr. D.C. Jarvis, in his excellent book on folk medicine,* points this out. All blood in the body passes through the thyroid where the gland secretes iodine to kill germs. The iodine content of the gland is dependent upon its intake of iodine in food.

Iodine has long been used as a folk remedy to quiet the nerves and relieve hypertension. Dr. Jarvis suggests that one drop of Lugols solution (a druggist may prepare this for it contains only five percent of elemental iodine in a ten percent solution of potassium iodide) Should be taken daily.

Citric Acid. The normal acid alkaline pH0 balance of the body chemistry is slightly acidic and should the urine demonstrate an alkaline pH on litmus paper then it may be assumed that a cold or some other disturbance is affecting the body's chemistry. The therapeutic procedure is to shift the chemistry back to the acid position as quickly as possible. The citric fruits are used to accomplish this. Hot lemonade is a first choice but any of

---

Arthritis and Folk Medicine. Published in 1960 by Fawcett, Crest Books, Greenwich, CT.

the citrus fruits, such as oranges, grapefruits, or limes, will suffice.

Facial pain is also associated with an alkaline urine reaction. Again citric acid or apple cider vinegar will relieve this pain. The suggested dosage is one teaspoon in a glass of water every hour for at least seven hours.

Vinegar. Dr Jarvis is strongly in favor of apple cider vinegar for the relief of many diseases. He recommends it for people suffering from arthritis. The suggested dosage is one tablespoon of vinegar and two of honey in a glass of water taken each day. Another benefit for the sufferer of arthritis who follows this suggestion—he will become calm and easier to live with.

Garlic. For years garlic was regularly prescribed for the treatment of high blood pressure and also the common cold. The author uses garlic capsules at the first sign of a cold and, as a result, hasn't had a cold in years. There is an offensive odor associated with the use of garlic, but this can be overcome by dissolving one or two chlorophyl tablets in the mouth right after swallowing the garlic.

Using revitalizing nutritives in the form of food instead of drug cures makes good sense. Every part of the body relies on proper nutrition to function well. Often the consumption of these vital food elements can help replace worn out tissue, promote resistance to infection, and assist organs and glands in operating more efficiently.

4 Holistic Hygiene: Environmental Influences

Many people are fond of ascribing their depressed spirits to the state of the weather. Understanding the influences that thermal and barometric pressure changes exert upon the human system may relieve people of much of the anxiety they experience in regard to their effects upon health.

Among the other holistic hygiene principles to be applied to your lifestyle are the following facts about temperature.

The average temperature of the air in the United States is fifty-five degrees Farenheit; the normal temperature of our bodies is ninety-eight degrees. Hence the average difference between the heat of the body and its environment is about forty-eight degrees. But the air temperature sometimes falls below zero, more than nature intended the body to be subjected to. It is the nature of heat to be forever seeking an equilibrium; hence all bodies, whether animate or inaminate, having a temperature above that of the atmosphere, tend to lose their excess heat. The speed with which an object loses heat depends on the amount of difference between the internal and external temperatures. The human body loses more heat in a given time than an inanimate object because it not only parts with its heat by radiation, like a stone, but also in other ways peculiar to living beings. The surface of the body is always moist, and evaporation of this moisture is a most potent cooling agent to the skin. The body also parts with its heat through the actions of several excretory organs, and a great deal is carried off by the large body of air which is constantly being warmed and expired from the lungs.

The loss of heat which the body is compelled to replenish is perpetual, but exceedingly variable in degree. The temperature of the atmosphere not only has its yearly and daily variations, but is subject to hourly and unexpected ones.

All atmospheric changes influence the system's vital and vito-chemical functioning. All parts of the body are pervaded by sensory nerves which receive impressions and convey them in every direction. When any part of the surface of the body receives an impression of external temperature, every part of the organism related to it in any way is immediately affected.

That function of the body which is directly related to external temperature is the heat-making process. Since the point of temperature at which vital actions take place is fixed, and since body heat is dependent upon its own resources, it follows that the production of body heat is accelerated or retarded to an extent exactly proportionate to the loss experienced.

This regulation of the body temperature is directly

related to the employment of the materials which are necessary to the production of vital phenomena. The system is thus relieved of any surplus of heat which it may have acquired by means of an increased evaporation from the surface, while the want of heat that is felt stimulates the respiratory organs into greater activity. To place the hand or foot, or any portion of the warm surface of the person, in contact with a very cold substance—such as a piece of ice—instantaneously causes an expansion of the ribs, a depression of the diaphragm, and consequently an unusually profound inspiration which is involuntarily continued until the heat that has been lost is fully restored. The heat of the body, or any part of it, may be depressed for a short time without any injury because it requires time for the physiological changes to complete their effects upon the economy.

In hot weather climates, such respiratory stimulus is less, respiration is consequently diminished, and the result is a retention of the materials that should be extruded from the system through the respiratory activity. When such materials are not completely reduced to carbonic acid, water and urea, the process is arrested and this results in state called biliousness, which suggests the presence of bile in the blood.

Importance of Cold. Invalids in particular are incapable of bearing the amount of cold suited to the respiratory needs of the average body. Many shrink from the very influence which would stimulate and invigorate their powers, instead repressing and cramping their already weakened faculties. The importance of developing the heat-making faculty is equal to that of exercise, and is among the first things about which the chronic invalid should be instructed.

The effect of cold is to infuse into the system an agreeable vigor; but in a weakened state of the system and perverted condition of the nerves the sensations, being abnormally acute, will often rebel. This indicates a need for discipline, the very process required to reinstate health. It is only when the withdrawal of heat from the system is not accompanied by a corresponding increase of respiration that exposure to cold can be hurtful; for it is then that refuse matter of the system is retained and conflicts with the vital processes.

Cold Bath. This may be either generally applied to the whole surface or locally, applied to some portion of the body. In either case the general effect is similar, though the particular side effects may widely differ. The first impression of ice cold water upon a part of the body acts through the sensory nerves, causing the ribs to expand and labored breathing to result . The respiratory condition continues so long as the body or any part of it is losing an unusual amount of heat; it continues until the equilibrium is restored.

The water coming in contact with the warm skin has acquired the body's heat, which is compensated by increased respiration. A sitting bath with the temperature elevated by two degrees, will have caused the absorption of oxygen by the blood from four or five cubic feet of air—enough to raise a half-pint of water from the freezing point to the boiling point—and will have eliminated from the system more than a half-ounce of solid material.

Warm Bath. When the temperature of the air is considerably below that of the body, we know that the body receives heat from it at only a very moderate rate; but the temperature of water does not feel warm to us until it approximates our own. At ninety-eight degrees it ceases to receive heat from us, and therefore when the body is submerged in a bath of that temperature, the ordinary incentive for the production of heat ceased to act and all the physiological processes are retarded. Respiration becomes slow and difficult and the system soon suffers from retained matters. If there has been pain, the bath affords a delightful sense of relief and may check the morbid action.

Hot Bath. In a bath of this type, heat is imparted to the body, which compels a reciprocal action to return to normal—the body thus producing moisture at the surface to be evaporated. The skin, under the influence of the heat, breaks out in perspiration proportionate to the temperature. The superficial capillaries fill with blood, and central portions of the body are consequently relieved of their engorgement. While this may provide temporary relief, such a reaction cannot continue for any length of time without serious detriment to the body.

The important and radical difference between the effects of cold and warm bathing is that cold baths, due to their effects on respiration, function as aids in the removal of solid materials from the body, while warm and hot baths assist the system in removing fluid and saline matters.

Compresses. These usually consist of linen or cotton cloth, several times folded, thoroughly wetted, and applied to some part of the body. If soaked in hot water, the application is called a fomentation. This is beneficial to a painful body part. If cold, it soon acquires the temperature of the body and produces an effect upon the parts analogous to that of a warm bath.

Wet compresses also supply the conditions for osmosis, the interchange of fluids between different structures of the body. They are useful in congestions because the absorption of fluid through the capillary walls into the vessels detaches the corpuscles, which in this case are apt to adhere to the walls. This aids the escape of the clogged blood from the point of congestion.

Air Bath. This consists of simply baring the body, and exposing it to the air or a fan. This may be continued for a moderate length of time and should be accompanied by light and rapid friction with the hands over the whole surface of the body. The rubbing necessitates useful bending and stretching of the body in all directions.

Shower and Water Jet Baths. These are highly useful as local applications, readily inducing derivative effects in visceral organs, and at the same time exerting the same general influence as has previously been described. The shower may be unfit for certain ill individuals as it may be too severe. A small jet stream may be more manageable and milder. In these baths, the effect on the skin of the running water is stimulating. In each case, any sudden application should be avoided, as it may prove harmful for the patient.

Light. The fact that light has powerful hygienic, even remedial, properties is often overlooked. Light is a chemical agent. It arouses the plant world into life and perfects its products; without it all animate life would soon perish for lack of sustenance. It is a determining agent for the chemical state or bodies, readily decomposing numerous chemical compounds and recombining their elements into new forms.

There are several sources of light, the sun being the most important. Certain organisms develop or not according to the kind of light to which they are exposed. Some people suffer when exposed to fluorescent light. This inexpensive form of light is produced by energy reacting on a gas. It fluctuates and this could be the problem. Some authorities say children in their classrooms have become hyperactive under fluorescent lights. Adults working in offices and factories have suffered aberrations working under fluorescent lighting. The numbers of individuals for whom this is a problem seems to be very small and the reasons for the adverse reactions have not yet been discovered.

5   Holistic Mental Health

A great many of those who are mentally ill complain that some particular emotional trouble, such as disappointment, or excitement of feeling, was the original cause of their state; but few think of looking for relief, or are led to look for it, in a restoration of order and harmony to the disturbed mind. Only a few seem to realize that the forces that exercise such potent control over the organism for the production of disease may be made equally available for the restoration of health! The ordinary practice of medicine instills the notion that the business of the physician is simply to supply and regulate certain conditions by means of pills, powders and solutions.

However, extraordinary states of the mind do result in extraordinary states of the physical body, and they can be wholesome or unwholesome. If the effects continue for any considerable length of time the consequences may be serious, even permanent. Some scientists believe that the continued indulgence of malicious feelings, for instance, will modify those internal functions of the system which serve to check disease and will finally overcome their vital power; thus any latent tendencies to chronic disease will be activated. Diseases are produced, if not perpetuated, by causes over which mere chemical influences cannot exercise any positive control. Headache, nervousness, heart disease, or dyspeptic problems may be indications of some peculiar morbid state of the mind or of the emotional state of the sufferer. In these cases, every medical prescription is totally irrelevant unless it recognizes the operation of causes existing in a sphere beyond the reach of the most potent drug. Fatal mistakes may result when the patient is advised to try the resources of an inexhaustible pharmacy instead of common sense!

The truth is, the influence of the mind over the body is as great in health as it is in disease. The influence of the body over the mind is equally true. The actions of the muscles influence the mind. An eighteenth century German writer Dr. Feuchersleben, wrote,

> "Who is unacquainted with the sparkling eye, the free respiration, the glowing color, and the serene brow of the joyous? Who is not familiar with the trembling aspect, the hesitating utterance, the cold ruffled skin, the bristling hair, the palpitating heart, the impeded respiration, the paleness, the low pulse, and the thousand other signs of fear? The slow oppressed breathing, interrupted by sobs, the cold, pallid, wrinkled skin, the slow tottering gait, and the weak pulse of the despairing? The deep broad blush of shame, or the pallor of miserable envy? The beaming countenance of requited love,

or the anguished expression of disappointed affection? The spasmodic constriction of throat and chest which accompanies jealousy? The gnawing pain which torments the heart of devilish hate? The storm in the veins of the angry man, his inflamed countenance, his gasping breath, his bounding pulse, and wild swollen countenance?"

All of these external manifestations depend upon certain changes effected by the mind. The extraordinary state into which the system is thrown soon subsides and the ordinary physical and mental conditions return and so the effects are not necessarily permanent. But if these conditions are continued for any considerable length of time, then the consequences may be serious, or even fatal.

The attending physican will encounter extraordinary difficulties in overcoming chronic states of disease by ordinary medicine when the disease is perpetuated, even produced, by causes not subject to chemical intervention. This fact may even be acknowledged by the physican but he usually cannot investigate the relationships or know how to make an investigation useful. He may even be unwilling to acknowledge that the headache, the nervousness, the heart disease or the dyspeptic condition which he is called upon to remedy are only indications of some particularly morbid state of the mind or of the emotional disturbance of the sufferer. In these cases the medical prescription must be totally irrelevent unless the perscription recognizes the operation of causes in a sphere beyond the reach of the most potent drug. What happens to the patient when the physician turns the patient over to the care of the pharmacist instead of using common sense to diagnose the disease? Can the physician be called a healer if he devotes his attention exclusively to the superficial and deceptive signs of disease and ignores the fact that the body is only the expression of the interior, of the invisible and imperishable spirit of the patient? Shouldn't the physician learn to heal by faith as well as by science?

Was this the secret of Anton Mesmer? Did he discover that the thoughts, feelings and mental habits of the patient needed rectifying as well as the chemistry of the body? It is a fact that a few physicians today talk about the physical effects of psychosomatic disease. They are beginning to suspect that a disease may not be less a disease because its source happens to lie in an unpredictable imagination or in excessive activity or in wrong modes of thought. People are beginning to see and understand the intangible causes of disease and to understand they are not incurable. But unfortunately medicine is not yet ready to give as much attention to the mental aspects and relations of disease as to the pulse, the tongue, the temperature of the skin, and the color and consistency of the excretions. Perhaps the physician doesn't know how to do this. You have probably been told by your doctor to slow down, that you are too tense, that you need to relax, that you need to get more rest. But he doesn't know how to accomplish these things himself, let alone tell you how, so he resorts to a chemical designed to regulate your body.

If you are a bundle of nerves he will, most likely,

prescribe a tranquilizer or a sleeping pill, or both. Relaxation is something that has to be learned and your doctor may know when but not how to prescribe relaxation.

Physical and mental relaxation work together. You can't have one without the other. You can't rest your body if your mind is in turmoil. You must slow down both mentally and physically. Every nerve impulse results in muscular contraction somewhere in your body and these contractions may be voluntary or involuntary. Contractions of the muscles of the neck may bring on a headache. Heart disease in relatively young people has been attributed to involuntary muscle contractions in the chest.

Psychogenic or psychosomatic illnesses originate in the mind or psyche and they take a heavy toll, one that seems to be ever-increasing, because there is a linkage between mankind and the ills of the world. Nervous fatigue, indigestion, disturbed sleep are seeds for disease. Most doctors do recognize this but can only suggest that the patient needs to change his ways and leave the procedure for change up to the patient.

A few years ago I recognized this need for a change in myself so I took up the game of golf. I wrongly thought that this change of pace would relax me. It did not. It was only a change in routine. The golf was stressful. In spite of my lessons I could never drive the ball the way I wanted to. I found out that for me this type of recreation was not true relaxation. Fortunately I was involved with hypnosis. I had already written several books on the

subject.* I knew how to enter a deep trance. Self-hypnosis became my tool for entering deep relaxation.

*Hypnotherapy and Troubled Children, Irvington Publishing Co., N.Y.C.
and New Horizon Press , N.J. How to Lose Weight and Stop Smoking
through Self-Hypnosis, Irvington Publishing Co. N.Y.C. Why Children
Fail, How to Help Them With Positive Suggestion, Irvington Publishing
Co. N.Y.C.

6 Holistic Principles of Self-Hypnosis and Yoga

Modern hypnosis is very different from the ancient meditative arts as practiced in the eighteenth century by James Esdaile and many others. The ancient healing art of "magnetism" or "mesmerism" is all but lost to the people of the twentieth century. Perhaps these ancient arts suggest black magic rather than scientific inquiry. A modern magnetic physican, if such a person exists, could be prosecuted for practicing medicine without a license even in the face of evidence amply demonstrating his prowess as a healer.

But the ancient art does live on under new names—cautiously, quietly and modestly. Today we do have transcendental meditation, laying-on of hands, yoga, Silva Mind Control, and so on. The term hypnosis is relatively new. It was coined by the nineteenth century English surgeon, James Braid, from a Greek word meaning "sleep"; but hypnosis is not sleep at all. For a while the meditative state was called the trance-umbra, which is a more appropiate term because it more accurately describes the state.

Self-hypnosis depends upon the individual's ability to get rid of tension and still the nerves. Tension is the great enemy of man. It exists on a conscious level as well as on a subconscious level. It creates fatigue and worry, defeats the individual's ability to concentrate, and contracts the muscles of the chest and the arteries leading to the brain.

Relaxation Technique

It is not appropriate for a doctor to tell a patient to relax because relaxation is an art that must be learned and takes practice to attain. It isn't learned overnight. Here is a technique that you can use to achieve deep relaxation:

1. First establish the time of day that is most convenient for your session. You may choose to do this as you arise in the morning or just before you retire at night.

2. Choose a time when you can be alone because it is harder to do this when other people are around. Later on, you will be able to relax anytime and anywhere.

3. Select a place where you can be quiet and where the noises of the neighborhood and home will least distract you.

4. Check your clothes. You shouldn't be aware of any article of clothing. The less you have on, the better it will be.

5. The room must be comfortable. If it is chilly or drafty, real relaxation will be impossible to achieve. I usually do this in my bedroom while wearing pajamas.

6. When you are ready, assume a comfortable posture and begin by taking at least ten deep breaths and then settle down to regular breathing.

7. Stretch one arm, relax; stretch the other arm, relax. Continue this stretching exercise until you have stretched and relaxed all four limbs.

8. Do it again.

9. Note the sensations within your body as you let go, for it is the process of letting go that you want to remember, both consciously as well as subconsciously. Letting go is the key to deep relaxation and it is something that has to be practiced.

10. Picture yourself as a puppet no longer supported by strings. There are no more strings holding you up so you relax completely. You can allow your body to become heavy and your mind can become drowsy.

11. You are now ready for what is called the progressive relaxation technique.

A. Think of a healing force coming down from the top of your head to the bottom of your feet. Consciously let go of the muscles in the scalp.

B. Let this feeling extend over your brow to your eyes. Think of your eyes feeling better, feeling stronger.

C. Let this feeling of deep relaxation extend down through the muscles of your face. Let go of the jaw muscles so that the mouth is just slightly ajar.

D. Think of this healing force moving down your arms—first one arm and then the other—and across your shoulders, down into your finger tips. You can shake your finger tips a little if you want to.

E. Think of this healing force going inside your chest

to relax the muscles around your heart. Picture your healthy heart and lungs. Breathing easily. Low blood pressure. You have never felt better in your life.

F. Picture your lungs and kidneys easily removing impurities so that you feel better and better.

G. Let this feeling of deep relaxation go down your spine. You will soon feel it tingle from the power of your deep concentration.

H. Think of this great healing power going down and into your stomach. Through your buttocks and on through your thighs.

I. Begin to feel the healing force, passing into your legs.

J. And lastly, think of your feet and of the healing force going into your toes.

12. When you join the progressive relaxation sequence with deep concentration you will find yourself on the edge of total drowsiness. Your mind and your body will arrive at a special state of consciousness, open to suggestions and open to examination. You will rest every part of your body to an even greater degree than in natural sleep.

The progressive relaxation sequence should take you no more than fifteen minutes. You can begin your day with suggestions to carry with you all day long. You can use the sequence in the middle of the day, if you can find a place where you can be alone for a few minutes, and give yourself a second wind to carry you through a busy afternoon schedule.

When the time comes to end your moments of deep relaxation, you should swiftly reverse the sequence and restore the muscle tone to each part of your body and then enjoy a luxurious stretch. Eventually you will be able to accomplish deep relaxation in the company of others. You can learn to do it in an airplane, as a passenger in an automobile, even in an office. Just close your eyes for a few minutes and think through the sequence and then arouse yourself, recharged and ready to tackle your responsibilities.

In many ways deep relaxation is superior to a nap or even to a longer sleep where the body tosses and turns throughout the night. The dreams and the continued contraction of the muscles during the night can leave the sleeper almost as tired as he was before going to sleep. Deep relaxation can do more for a tired individual in just a few minutes than hours of fitful sleep.

Deep relaxation is the forerunner to the more advanced state of meditation that is popularly termed self-hypnosis. This is the first step in shutting out all flittering thoughts, all the mental garbage, to allow the thinking process to concentrate its efforts upon one central and chosen thought. This is the final step in mental and physical healing.

Concentration Technique

Most people have become helpless slaves to the mental and physical storms that surround them. They are attracted and manipulated by external stimuli over which they have no control; as a result they cannot purposely pursue a single goal. Their energies are consumed by distractions, and so their goals constantly elude them.

Many of these hapless people spend hours, weeks and even years disciplining their bodies, but neglect to train their minds. But their minds are the keys to the perfection they desire. The interrelationships between the mind and the body require this effort because these two facets of the human being are not divisible. Here is one way to train your mind:

1. The first thing to do as you begin the first lesson is to select an image upon which to focus your attention. This can be anything close at hand. Try to think of this one object for ten seconds, then twenty seconds, then thirty seconds, forty seconds and so on. The important thing is to prevent the mind from wandering. This is your first mental exercise.

If you like, you can shut your eyes as you concentrate and if the image you are concentrating upon fades, open them to refresh your image. Eventually you will be able to maintain a mental picture and the correlating benefit will be the development of the ability to bar uninvited distractions and disruptions from your mental processes. You will be able to listen better to other people. Your decision-making will improve. You will be able to acquire knowledge faster and you will retain what you have learned.

2. During your periods of concentration, empty your mind of irritating thoughts. Your goal is peace of mind; let go of all your worries. Emotions of any kind must not interfere with your concentration. You will learn to shut out all thoughts except the ones you want to entertain. The instant a daydream tries to come in, drive it out. You will be pleasantly surprised to see how quickly you learn the act of concentration

3. There are special benefits available to those who practice concentration in the evening. You can go to sleep with the concentrated thought in your mind. At night while you are asleep, your mind will continue to function so that, in the morning, you will awaken with some fresh thoughts about the subject. You may find solutions to difficult problems while you sleep.

4. The key thought in meditation is *let go*, but don't make the mistake of trying to force unwanted thoughts out of your mind; just let them go. I use a burning candle during my hypnosis seminars as a focal point for the members of the class. I also use a candle for individuals who come to my office for training in self-hypnosis. I ask my subjects to concentrate upon the flame. I ask them to think about the flame—to examine the colors, the movements and to consider all of its attributes. They are told to close their eyes and visualize the flame. Should the visualization fade away, they are to reopen their eyes to look again at the flame until, at last, they can hold the visualized flame in their mind's eyes.

5. Concentration such as I have just described is the key to examining yourself. You can learn to question your motives. You will enjoy the sense of freedom that comes when you can separate yourself from your immediate environment. You can examine your thoughts and actions by separating from them and becoming your own psychologist.

You can really change your character by changing the way you think. You can find peace of mind when you free yourself from anger, resentment and hate.

6. Highly placed among the desirable attributes of con-

centration power is an improved memory. A poor memory usually exists because the individual can't focus his attention upon anything long enough for an impression to be made. Except in the most unusual of instances, a good memory is developed through training.

Memory Improvement Techniques

There are a number of exercises to develop your memory:

A. After leaving a room, mentally review the number of items in it.

B. In the evening, just before you go to sleep, review all of your day's activities. Go to sleep thinking of ways to improve yourself, your motives, your handling of situations.

C. Take a deck of cards and deal yourself five of them. After you have examined the five cards, turn them over and recall them. Examine them again to check your memory of them. When you can successfully remember five cards go on to six, then seven, then eight and so on until you can recall the entire deck.

D. You will learn to direct the hidden power of your mind, to heal physical as well emotional problems. After all, your mind is directly linked to every area of your body. You can really get sick by just thinking about illness. It follows that you can get well by thinking positively.

A great many people, upon reading a book about diseases, think of the symptoms and relate them to their own bodies. As they consider the diseases they have been reading about, they tend to take on some of the symptoms. You can consciously counteract unconscious impulses to feel sick and begin to feel well.

E. Even many serious illnesses take root in emotional problems and poor mental attitudes. Problems of the back, arthritis and other diseases related to stress can seldom be alleviated by drugs alone. A physican may be able to alleviate the pain, but the disease will remain as long as the patient keeps the same old negative attitudes

The hidden power of concentration contains the key to unlock many diseases. It enables the patient to complement the physicans work, to overcome many diseases. And the best part about it is that it doesn't cost a penny.

Meditation Technique

Meditation is really self-hypnosis. The first step toward this is to learn how to concentrate. Meditation allows the individual to analyze himself objectively.

Self-analysis, if it is to have real meaning to an individual, doesn't involve self-pity, guilty feelings or New Year's resolutions to mend or change ways of behavior. Self-analysis is an honest appraisal of an individual's way of thinking about himself and others and what has been done and said. Self-analysis involves getting rid of mental garbage, superficial and incorrect personal assessments, and negative, hostile attitudes.

Self-analysis involves the selection of problems to be resolved, changed, or accepted and lived with. Self-analysis through self-hypnosis requires the individual to concentrate long enough upon a single thought and to be able to examine that thought very carefully. While doing so he must keep self-excuses, self-deprecation, self-guilt, self-doubt out of his mind. It is easy to find excuses, escapes and camouflages for evading responsibility and the truth. Self-analysis through self-hypnosis can enable the individual to re-educate himself and redirect his energies along the constructive avenues open to him.

Here are some steps that will direct you into meditation:

1. As a beginner you must find some place where you can be alone. Close the door to your room and, if necessary, take the telephone off the hook. You can't meditate if you are vulnerable to any kind of interruption.

2. It is best to practice early in the morning or after every one else has gone to bed and to follow the same routine daily for at least two weeks.

3. You need to make yourself as comfortable as possible, so wear clothing that cannot bind you in any way. It is hard to concentrate if your belt, tie or shoes are constricting you.

4. Your room should be free of glaring lights as well obtrusive sounds. If you can't find a a suitable place in your own home, you might try the reading room in your local library. A page in one of their books might serve as the object of your concentration.

5. When you are ready, assume a comfortable posture and look steadily at the object that you have selected. It can be a word in a book, a figure in a picture or even, as I have done while sitting on a beach, a distant sailboat.

6. Concentrate upon the object until everything else fades from your vision. When this happens, move all your thoughts to the object. When you have succeded in letting go of all outward thoughts you will be in a state of self-hypnosis.

Self-hypnosis is a skill that must be learned. It just doesn't come automatically; it is an acquired skill and one worth having. You don't have to select a picture or an object. A thought will do just as well. You can select a religious thought or symbol; you can select a part of your body, your heart or lungs. When you are concentrating, consider every detail of the subject—its composition, variations, color, function, rhythms, vistas, etc. When I use a candle as part my lectures or in the office, I ask my subjects to consider every aspect of the flame—to consider spiritual connotations: enlightment, the light of the world, warmth, symbolism and individuals who have shed light upon the world. The added benefit for meditation of this kind is that it opens up the individual to self-analysis. It develops insight and encourages a disentanglement from daily problems. It frees the mind from inner prisons, fears, failures and self-destructive thoughts.

Re-education made possible though self-hypnosis frees the mind from dwelling upon past mistakes and failures and encourages consideration of the successful experiences, that seem to get overlooked. Success is the mother of additional successes in the same way that failure, when dwelt upon, is the mother of additional failure.

Self-Hypnosis Technique

Let me present a few of the principles of the art of self-hypnosis. Find a quiet place where you can be alone—where you can relax mentally as well as physically—and then count the ten deep breaths. You already know how to do this from the relaxation technique given in chapter 6.

Relax and begin self-hypnosis. You have practiced this before. You know how it feels to be completely relaxed with your body, mind and spirit in perfect harmony. Permit your human trinity of body, mind, and spirit to completely relax. Use your imagination and take yourself back to some special place where you have found peace in the past or in your imagination. Was it a beach where you reclined on the sand? You were completely warm and the summer breeze was gentle upon your body. You listened to the soft music that wavelets made—coming and going, rolling sand along the beach. The soft summer breeze caressed you and you relaxed and felt at peace in your lovely private place. You watched the soft summer clouds drift slowly by. You seemed to be drifting along with them. Let go of the present time and feel free to drift into another level of consciousness. Don't hold yourself back; let yourself go into relaxation—free of tensions, free of anxieties, completely comfortable with your triune existence. All of your tensions are leaving as you relax and meditate. Rest deeply and go still deeper into this meditative state where you are finding freedom from cares. There is nothing that can disturb you while you are in deep meditation. Take ten deep breaths:

One.   Relax and inhale. As you inhale, go deeper and deeper into relaxation.

Two.   Take another deep breath. Inhale and then exhale deeper and deeper.

Three.   Take a deep breath, deep, deep, and deeper.

Four.   Take another deep breath and then let it all go. Go deeper and deeper into relaxation.

Five.   Inhale and then exhale. Go deeper and deeper into relaxation.

Six.   Inhale and then exhale again and go deeper and deeper into relaxation. Release your consciousness and permit yourself to let go.

Seven.   Take another deep, deep breath and let yourself relax more deeply. Release your conscious control. Don't hold back.

Eight.   Inhale another deep, deep, deep breath. You are about to go deeper and deeper into self-hypnosis than you have ever been before.

Nine.   Take another deep breath and go deeper and deeper into hypnosis.

Ten.   Take still another deep, deep breath and let yourself go into deep relaxation.

At this point you can test your hypnotic state, as described in the Weight Control Meditation section in chapter 7, or you can go right along with the meditation message. Remember, you can learn to enter hypnosis anytime you want to; and don't worry about waking up because that is the easy part.

You can make your own arousal sequence or simply

say, "I am now going to wake myself up. I am going to
count to five, and at the count of five I will be wide
awake, feeling really good about myself.

One.   I am waking up, feeling good.
Two.   I feel very good and I am coming up, out of
            my trance.
Three.   I am waking up now, feeling fine.
Four.   I am waking up, feeling better and better
            about myself.
Five.   Wake up! Wake up! Wake up!

Yoga

Yoga is a health practice developed several thousand
years ago. Some people confuse it with religion or some
kind of philosophy but it is neither of these. It can make
almost magical improvements in the emotional and physical health of any individual willing to invest a considerable amount of time in its study.

I had been a student of hypnosis for forty years before
discovering yoga.* I was amazed to discover that many
of my hypnotic procedures had come from yoga.

It is interesting to note that the modern hypnotist and
the ancient practioners of yoga approach the meditative
state in the same ways, except for posture. The yogis
prefer a sitting position. I usually meditate in bed, just
before arising in the morning. I have tried all of the
classic sitting positions, but prefer the prone position.

*Yoga. Desmond Dunne. Wilfred Funk Publishers N.Y.C. 1953

One reason given by the proponents of yoga for using a sitting position while meditating is the tendency of some meditating individuals to drift off into a sleep state. This tendency would negate the meditative effort. If you have a tendency to fall asleep while meditating, then you should try a sitting position but you may find a comfortable chair more relaxing than the cross-legged sitting position prescribed in yoga. The most advanced of these, the lotus pose, does have physical value. Because it is a stretching position it will limber up the joints and muscles of the legs and even the hips. However, some individuals out of condition may need time and more practice before they are able to achieve the full lotus pose.

I have already pointed out that the mind and body are part of an organic whole. What affects one affects the other, directly or indirectly. Therefore, emotional tensions can cause a physical illness. The opposite is just as true; a relaxed mental condition cures a physical illness brought on by tension. A relaxed mind and body are essential for well-being. Yoga is a way to accomplish this goal. It can't stop the aging process, but it does slow it down by improving the metabolism, muscle tone, skin tone, elimination, vitality and vigor, and appetite.

There is no magic formula or an elixir of youth. To search for it is a waste of time. Beauty will fade; physical prowess will diminish. But yoga does promise a longer useful life—free of pain, weakness and other miseries of old age. This is what man really wants in this life, as Hindu sages discovered thousands of years ago.

7   Holistic Weight Control

You are overweight if you exceed the average weight for your body frame. Some people appear to have been destined to become overweight, having acquired their excess weight early in life. Maybe some of them were crying babies who were pacified frequently with bottles of milk and, as a result of the extra nourishment they received, they may have acquired a propensity toward obesity. This became their lifestyle. Unfortunately, fat children usually become fat adults.

For some people who have been fat most of their lives, dieting only seems to provide an interval of slimness between fat periods. The dieter perceives himself as fat, and during his slim phase continues to perceive himself as fat. He considers slimness as simply a temporary affair. He expects to return to fatness. In fact, he may even be uncomfortable while nervously waiting for the "inevitable fat" to return.

Eating, for some people, serves as a palliative for the emotional problems they encounter. When they are faced with a crisis or loneliness, they stuff themselves —food seems to relieve their bodily distress; they eat to salve their emotional hunger. This behavior dominates their eating habits. Eventually they may lose control over their eating habits altogether and not even realize how much food they consume.

According to the Metropolitan Life Insurance Company, there may be an inherent predisposition toward obesity in some people, just as there are inherent predispositions toward some emotional and physical dysfunctions with other people. Fat parents tend to have fat children. Why? Is this an inherited trait, or do these children simply learn their eating habits from their parents? The answer is not definitive. We do know that different people's bodies metabolize excess calories in different ways. Some people turn their excess calories immediately into heat, while others store them away for future use. The basal metabolism procedure varies infinitely from one individual to another.

Undoubtedly, a glandular dysfunction can account for a few cases of obesity. But if that's the cause, then obesity will not be the only symptom of the dysfunction. Other symptoms will overshadow the obesity symptom. Should you suspect that your weight problem is of glandular orientation, then you should immediately consult your medical doctor. In such cases undertaking an unsupervised diet is probably the worst thing you can do in attempting to overcome your weight . However, medical causes for obesity are rare. The common cause of obesity is overeating; and if overeating is coupled with a sedentary lifestyle, then the excess calories will be stored as fat. I would like to caution overweight people who have adopted a sedentary lifestyle not to suddenly embark upon a vigorous physical exercise program in a frantic effort to burn off excess calories or stored up fat. You may endanger your life! Fat is a hazard to exercise. You should consider intense physical conditioning only after your weight is normalized. Begin slowly.

Are you eating just as much now as you did when you were a teenager . . . when you were growing and exercising and had the benefits of a faster metabolism? If you have grown older and have slowed down, then you should eat less. If you are middle-aged and are overweight, you should reduce your caloric intake. It might even be critical that you do so. You have to change your eating habits. Self-hypnosis will make that an easy task for you to accomplish.

Your eating habits were established early in your life, but your changed lifestyle may have changed your diet so that it now includes richer—and consequently more fattening—foods. Do you remember something about the essential basic four food groups from elementary school? If your school was a typical one, then you were properly instructed about a "balanced diet." You were taught to eat something from the "basic four food groups" every day so that you would stay healthy.

In order to stay healthy, you were instructed to select at least one food from each of the basic groups every day. That's fine, but you may need to cut down on calorie intake as well. You may need to cut down your portions if you are gaining weight. Be sure to remember that the gravies and the sauces that you put on your foods can contain just as many calories as the food itself.

You should be sure to see a reputable medical doctor

1. Milk Group   Whole, skim, evaporated, instant, non-fat dry, buttermilk, with cheese or ice cream as alternates.
Adults .... 1 cup
Children .... 3–4 cups

2. Meat Group   2 to 3 ounces of lean, cooked meat, poultry or fish; 2 eggs; 1 cup of dried beans, 4 tablespoons of peanut butter. Two or more servings.

3. Vegetable/
Fruit Group   A citrus fruit or other vitamin C fruit or vegetable daily. A dark, leafy green or deep yellow vegetable for vitamin A every other day. Other fruits and vegetables and potatoes every day. Two or three servings (a serving equals ½ cup).

4. Bread/Cereal
Group   Whole or enriched grain. Four or more servings. A serving is 1 slice of bread; 1 ounce of ready-to-eat cereal and ½ to ¾ cup of cooked cereal, noodles or rice.

(From Scott, Foresman, *Health and Your Health*, K–8, Glenview, IL) if you suspect that you have a metabolism problem that is causing you to gain weight. If you think, however, that your weight problem exists because you consume too many calories, then you should carefully plan a reducing diet. Of course, you need to know the caloric values of foods in order to do this. The best part of planning your own diet is that you will be able to select those foods that you like best.

WEIGHT LOSS THROUGH SELF-HYPNOSIS

If you need to change your eating habits, self-hypnosis is the best technique available to help accomplish this goal. For most people, overeating is an addiction that can be managed with hypnotherapy. This addiction is frequently caused by a psychological problem. Yet, even though the overeater may already have overcome that psychological problem, the overeating usually continues. This means that the overeater has developed a secondary problem—one that may be harder to overcome than the primary one.

Through the technique I suggest, you will be able to change your eating habits. You will not need a special diet to control your weight. Instead, you begin your new lifestyle by preparing a list of foods that you are now eating which are causing you to gain weight. Call this your negative list. Make another list of foods that are important for good nutrition and are not fattening. Call this your positive list.

While you are writing these lists, it would be a good

idea to write down some of your reasons for wanting to become slender. Here are some reasons you can add to your own suggestions for guiding your subconscious mind to work with you in becoming slender. First, do you have a family? If you do, then you will want to live as long as you can in order to be with them as long as you can. You are more apt to do this if you are slender. Second, are you seeking someone's love? You are more apt to be successful if you are slender because you will feel more desirable. You will also look better. You can't feel your best if you are overweight. With the addition of your own reasons your hypnotherapy becomes a personal thing.

If you have some unique reasons for changing your eating habits in order to become slender, you are going to send those reasons to your subconscious mind and use self-hypnosis in order to do it. You are going to tell your subconscious mind that you will enjoy food more by eating less. A bad habit that causes most obese people a lot of trouble is eating between meals. This habit may be a problem for you, but it is one that you can handle. Simply suggest to yourself, "I enjoy eating so much at the right times that I don't want to spoil my meals by eating between them. Besides, I no longer enjoy eating candy, cakes, etc." However, if you do encounter a lot of difficulty in overcoming the eating-between-meals habit, you may have to substitute something between your meal that is non-fattening. Apples might do nicely, as might such raw vegetables as celery or carrots.

Review all of your hypnotherapy goals as well as your motivations. Keep a mental picture before your mind's

eye and see yourself as a slender person. Re-examine
your emotional problems. If you do things that seem to
be causing you to overeat excessively, then use your
positive hypnotherapy suggestions to eliminate or modify
those things. Set a realistic weight loss goal for yourself
and don't get upset if you backslide and gain a few pounds
from time to time. Everybody does! You may lose a few
battles in your war against obesity, but you will win the
war if you are persistent.

Weight Control Meditation Tape

Practice the body relaxing and healing movements
mentioned in this book. Become conscious of the physical
differences that exist between body tension and body
relaxation. The physical movements will help you get
ready to enter a relaxed mental state. You have learned
that a comfortable physical setting for meditation (hypnotherapy) is critical while learning the art, but later
on—when you are experienced—just about any place
will do.

You can make your own hypnotherapy tape that will
augment this weight loss section of the book, using the
following words as though they were your own. As you
listen to the tape, try to empathize with it. Don't just
passively listen to it. Take each one of the deep breaths
as suggested on the tape. Continue using the tape, all
the self-improvement opportunities you desire will open
up to you. You will be at the threshold of a new, slimmer
life.

Practice the body relaxing movements and become ready to enter an equally relaxed mental state. Close your eyes and let your imagination take over while you dream of some special place where you have relaxed the hours away. Perhaps your special place was a quiet, secluded beach. Were you there in the afternoon when the sun was going down? Did you fall asleep while resting on the sand, still warm from the sun? The only sound that you could hear was the soft flowing music of waves rippling and rolling sand along the beach. The soft summer breeze caressed your body and you felt at peace with yourself while resting in your special place, watching the soft clouds drift by. You seemed to be drifting along with them. You let go of your consciousness. Don't hold onto it now! Begin to feel as free as the clouds you watched drift by. Your cares are beginning to leave you, and you are beginning to rest just as though you were back in your lovely, private place. You almost can hear the soft music of those waves rolling along the beach.

You are going to count to ten. With each count you are to take deep, relaxing breaths as you go deeper and deeper into this wonderful condition where you can free yourself of anxieties. There is nothing that can disturb you while you are in this meditative state.

One.	Breathe deeper and deeper. You are going to feel relaxed all through your body, your mind and your spirit.
Two.	Breathe more deeply than you did before and go deeper and deeper into relaxation.
Three.	Go deeper and deeper into relaxation with

each breath that you take. You are beginning
to feel very relaxed.

Four.   There is nothing to hold you back from deep
meditation. So, take a deep, deep breath and
let yourself go.

Five.   You are going to take another very deep
breath and drift deeper and deeper into the
most relaxed state that you have ever known.
Release your consciousness now.

Six.   Take still another deep, deep breath. You
are beginning to feel drowsy as you release
all of your anxieties. You can accomplish all
of your goals in hypnotherapy.

Seven.   Take another deep breath and relax your
mind, body and spirit. There is nothing that
can stop you from freeing yourself of every
anxiety and every tension

Eight.   Take still another deep breath and release
yourself. You are beginning to feel very
drowsy.

Nine.   Take another very deep breath and allow
yourself to drift off into the most relaxed state
you have ever known.

Ten.   Take just one more deep, deep, breath and
go into relaxation. Your eyes are closed and
they are very heavy. You are ready to allow
sleep to come.

Here is how you can deepen your trance. All you have
to say is, "I am going deeper and deeper asleep." Continue with:

One.	My eyes are getting heavy.
Two.	My eyes are getting heavy and I am closing them tighter and tighter.
Three.	My eyes are closed and they are locking together.

You can test your deepened hypnosis by counting to three. At the count of three you are to think, "I am going to swallow once, just once." Now let's count:

One.	My mouth is getting dry.
Two.	My mouth is getting drier and drier and I need to swallow.
Three.	I have to swallow now.

Feel yourself swallowing and realize that you are ready for post-hypnotic suggestions:

I am going to lose weight. In order to do this I will have to change my eating habits. I know that rich pastries, cake, candy and ice cream are all fattening, so I will eat protein foods instead. I will read over my "positive list" three times a day and substitute positive for negative nutrition whenever I am hungry. My reasons for wanting to be slender include these: I want to live longer, and I will if I am slender; I will look better; I will be more desirable when I am slender; I will feel better when I am slender, so I will eat less. I will enjoy food more by eating slowly and less. I will eat regular meals, composed of foods on my positive list. The less I eat, the better my food tastes. The less I snack, the more weight I lose. It's wonderful to control my eating habits and to watch the pounds of fat melt away. Losing weight is really easy. There is nothing to it.

Now it is time to arouse yourself:

One.   In a moment I will be wide awake.
Two.   I am beginning to wake up now and I feel fine.
Three.   I am waking up more and more.
Four.   My eyes are opening wide and I am waking up. Right Now!
Five.   Wake up! Wake up! Wake up!

Believe in yourself! Weight control takes time and effort, but self-hypnosis gives you will power. It's worth it! *You are worth it!*

The Holistic Diet Plan

Here is a new diet which is not a diet, but an improved lifestyle program. It is based on the affirmative values which your self-hypnosis program will create. Begin today! Choose positive instead of negative calories. The pounds will slip away and so will your old, bad habits. Conditioning is the key. Read over this list morning and evening. Live holistically and create the new you!
Unlike other diets, eating holistically takes into account

individual tastes and preferences. In order to follow this plan, you must accent the positive and delete negative choices. Hypnosis and meditation will help you stick to your new lifestyle. Make a list of the foods your family or you enjoy and then formulate a meal plan for the week using the positive choices on our chart. At first, do not try to count calories, but if you reach a plateau or choose to lose weight more quickly, begin to reduce your portions: first by one-third, then by one-half. Include snacks in your daily food proposals *but* positive not negative snacks. Very soon you will realize that you have formulated a new foodstyle. If you will add an exercise and meditative program to this nutritive one, you will be on your way to living holistically. Do not expect to accomplish your objective overnight. You did not gain weight or become flabby within twenty-four hours. Set small goals on your way to your ultimate aim. Reward yourself each time you reach these intermediate goals. These rewards should not be in the form of food but rather other tangible goods. When, through hypnosis, you can accept that food will no longer be counted as a reward since it does not accomplish but rather detracts from your real desires, then you will have an added incentive to stick to the holistic way of life. Ultimately, your new image will be the one you want to achieve—the one for which you have been searching without success.

*Positive vs Negative Diet Chart**

MEAL CHOICES

BEEF

Positive	Calories	Negative	Calories
Boiled, 3 oz.	185	Hamburger, 3 oz.	245
Lean Roast, 3 oz.	110	Short Ribs, 4 oz.	485
Lean Pot Roast	115	Stew Meat (Chuck)	505
Corned, Boiled	100	Suet	846
Round	197	Stew Meat (Round)	310

PORK

Positive	Calories	Negative	Calories
Simmered, lean	120	Simmered, fat	355
Chops, lean	120	Chops, fat	295
Roast, lean	160	Roast, fat	340
Spare Ribs (3) (Broiled)	123	Sausage	260
Shoulder (Broiled)	160	Picnic Ham Steak	246
		Tenderloin	287

LIVER

Positive	Calories	Negative	Calories
Calf, broiled	160	Calf, fried	222
Chicken, broiled (ea.)	50	Chicken, fried (ea.)	150
Beef, broiled	180	Beef, fried (4 oz.)	280

*Diet Chart by Nicole Nestel

CHICKEN

Positive	Calories	Negative	Calories
Broiled	100	Fried	325
Boiled	100	A la King	375
Chow Mein	125	Chicken Pie	350
Giblets	150	Cacciatore	550
Light (skinned, roasted)	155	Chop Suey	275
		Pot Pie	350
Dark (skinned, roasted)	157	Creamed Chicken	375
		Curried Chicken	325

TURKEY

Positive	Calories	Negative	Calories
Roast (1 slice)	100	Creamed	430
Smoked	125	Hashed	300
Lean, light roasted (3 oz.)	150	Potted	272
		Roasted (4 oz.)	305
Lean, dark roasted (3 oz.)	173		

FISH

Positive	Calories	Negative	Calories
Flounder, baked	71	Fishsticks (4½ oz.)	276
Sole, broiled	100	Mackerel, salted	305
Salmon, broiled	140	Mackerel, broiled	225
Shad, broiled	125	Shad Roe	362
Scallop, broiled	112	Scallops, fried	194
Bass	100	Bluefish, fried	325
Bluefish, broiled	185	Tuna (canned in oil)	288
Tuna (canned in water)	110	Creamed Oyster Stew	200
Codfish	100	Whitefish, smoked	180
,Whitefish, steamed	115	New England Clam Chowder	203
Manhattan Clam Chowder	85	Curried Fish	225
		Fish Chowder	210
		Lobster Bisque	200
		Vichyssoise	275

Meal Choices, (Continued)

SHELLFISH

Positive	Calories	Negative	Calories
Baked Oysters (12)	85	Oyster Stew w/milk	
Blue Point Oysters (12)	100	(1 cup)	200
Raw Oysters on the		Oysters, fried (12)	500
Half Shell (12)	100	Oysters Rockefeller	
Cherrystones (12)	125	(12)	360
Clams, steamed (12)	100	Stuffed Deviled Clams	200
Shrimp (12)	120	Clams, fried (12)	400
Shrimp Cocktail (12)	150	Shrimp Creole (12)	340
Lobster Cocktail,		Shrimp, fried (12)	240
½ cup	90	Lobster Newburg	185
Lobster, canned	100	Broiled Lobster	
Broiled Lobster	150	w/butter	250

EGGS

Boiled	75	Fried	100
Poached	75	Deviled	175
Coddled	75	Creole	200
Shirred	75	Scrambled w/milk	300
Egg Drop Soup	60	Creamed Egg	
		Sandwich w/butter	350

VEGETABLES & FRUITS (also for snacks)

Apple	75	Apple Pie	275
Dried Apricot (1½)	50	Apricot Mousse	350
Banana	100	Banana Split	450
Blackberries (fresh or		Blackberry Pie	350
water-packed, 1		Cherry Pie	350
cup)	100	Cherry Ice Cream	150
Cantaloupe (½)	50	Grapefruit, canned	75
Cherries, fresh (25)	75	Grapes (Malay,	
Grapefruit (½)	50	Muscat, Tokay)	100

Positive	Calories	Negative	Calories
Grapes (Concord	85	Orange Chiffon Pie	350
Delaware Niag-		Pineapple, canned	200
ara)	75	Pineapple Ices	100
Orange	75	Raspberry Ice	100
Pineapple, fresh		Raspberry Pie	350
(1 cup)	75	Strawberries,	
Pineapple, canned		(canned)	225
(1 slice)	50	Strawberry Sundae	400
Raspberries, fresh	50	Artichoke, stuffed	
Raspberries, canned	100	w/mushrooms and	100
Strawberries, fresh	50	breadcrumbs	
Strawberries, fro-		Artichoke, Jerusa-	80
zen	115	lem, raw	200
Artichoke (1)	75	w/butter sauce	
Artichoke Heart (1)	50	Asparagus Souffle	790
Asparagus (12)	25	Dried Kidney Beans	150
Mung Sprouts (1		(1 cup)	200
cup)	20	Lima Beans (1 cup)	
Soy Sprouts (1 cup)	50	Navy Beans (1 cup)	700
String Beans	25	Dried Navy Beans	230
Yellow Beans	25	(1 cup)	200
Snap Beans	25	Soy Beans (1 cup)	225
Potato, baked	125	Creamed Corn	
Potato, boiled	125	Potatoes Au Gratin	250
Sweet potato, boiled	210	Potatoes, browned	
Potato mashed	180	in	155
Broccoli, raw	45	butter	
Cabbage, raw	20	Potatoes, French	300
Eggplant	50	fried (10)	450
Green Pepper	25	Candied Sweet	50
Squash, summer	35	Potato	150
Squash, butternut	35	Sweet Potato Pie	600
Spinach	25	Broccoli, baked	125
Tomatoes	25	Broccoli, stuffed	100
Squash, hubbard	50		

Meal Choices (Continued)

GRAINS

Positive	Calories	Negative	Calories
Cracked Wheat Bread	60	Banana Bread	135
French Bread	55	Boston Brown Bread	140
Gluten Bread	35	Bran Raisin Bread	145
Graham Bread	55	Corn Bread	130
Rye Light Bread	55	Gingerbread	180
Whole Wheat Bread	55	Spoon Bread	199
Melba Toast	25	Cinnamon Bread	130
Puffed Wheat Cereal, unsweetened	54	Puffed Wheat Cereal, sweetened	132
Puffed Rice Cereal, unsweetened	60	Puffed Rice Cereal, sweetened	175
Wheat Germ, toasted	23	Frosted Flakes	147
Rice, precooked instant	180	Rice, white long-grain	223

DAIRY PRODUCTS

Positive	Calories	Negative	Calories
Skim Milk, 1 cup	88	Whole Milk, 1 cup	159
Half & Half, 1 cup	324	Heavy Cream, 1 cup	838
Yogurt, plain, 8 oz.	150	Sour Cream, 8 oz.	432
Whipped Butter, 1 cup	1081	Stick Butter, 1 cup	1625
Cottage Cheese, dry curd, 1 cup	125	Cottage Cheese, creamed large curd	239
Mozzarella Cheese (1 oz)	79	Blue Cheese (1 oz)	104
Camembert Cheese (1 oz)	85	Swiss Cheese (1 oz)	105
Muenster Cheese (1 oz)	85	Cheddar Cheese (1 oz)	113
Frozen Yogurt, plain 1 cup	180	Frozen Custard 1 cup	334
Ice Milk, 5.1% fat 1 cup	199	Ice Cream, fat, 1 cup	329

Snack Choices

DRINKS

Positive	Calories	Negative	Calories
Apple Cider	100	Apple Juice	125
Orange Juice		Orange Juice	
(unsweetened)	55	(sweetened)	75
Tomato Juice	40	Pineapple	125
Lemon	30	Apricot	120
Carrot	50	Nectarine	100

NUTS

Pistachio (16)	50	Brazil (5)	250
Peanuts (5)	53	Walnuts (10)	130
Litchi (10)	63	Butter (5)	200

MISCELLANEOUS

Dill Pickle	15	Potato Chips	158
Pretzel Sticks (10)	23	Brownie (1)	120
Rye Krisp (5)	30	Butterscotch	114
Sugar Wafer (1)	15	Popcorn, buttered	150
Popcorn, plain	50	Corn Chips	156
Gingersnap	20	Peanut Butter (2 tsp.)	200
Oyster Crackers	43	Short Cake	350
Cheese Crackers	15		
Pretzel Twists	58		
Angel Food Cake			
(1 slice)	110		
Pound Cake			
(1 slice)	130		

8 Holistic Therapy for Nervous Disorders

The suffering of many chronically ill individuals, especially those afflicted with disorders of the digestive system, generally consists, not so much of absolute pain, as of a peculiar and somewhat indefinite unhealthy sensation which, for want of a better term, they call nervousness.

Nervousness is apt to be considered a trivial symptom. However, if it is regarded in conjunction with the real suffering experienced by the invalid or to the permanent nature of the illness, it must be admitted to be one of the most serious of the symptoms.

Some nervous symptoms may be attributed to imperfect nutrition of the centers, where all nerve-force orginates. This, in turn, is dependent upon the other physiological functions whose work is to maintain the delicate balance among the general nutritive processes of the body.

Nervous symptoms exist in many degrees of intensity, even within the same person; sometimes they can arise because of depressed or irregular or greatly heightened functional actions of the nerve-centers. The impressions which these centers receive affect the consciousness, at times to a degree greatly beyond that to which the individual is accustomed. This may not, however, be due to the physiological state of the centers themselves, but in many cases to the generally poor condition of the whole system.

Unfortunately what follows is that the state of the nervous system, and consequently the mind, influences the body's physiological condition in such a way as to perpetuate this condition—in spite of all attempted medical treatments. In the opinion of the suffering individual there is nothing more important than the senses. And these senses being altered, he is constantly inclined to make improper choices to satisfy his wants and rectify his disorders—he eats improperly, drinks improperly, acts improperly—because his nerves are giving inaccurate signals.

Imperfection in the various nutritive actions is another common cause of nervous disorders. This subject will be dealt with more thoroughly later on. However, nervous diseases do not often occur in the absence of nervous abuse.

One class of causes to affect the sensory nerves and those of organic life are those brought on by the consuming of improper substances. The habitual use of pungent seasonings and beverages, which are stimulating and temporarily refreshing but not nutritious, is a common method of abusing the nerves. The organic needs of the system demand materials that are strictly nutritive; however, many ill people are unable to give the needed attention to this aspect of their environment.

Another cause of nervous disorders, and perhaps as important as any other, is medication in general. The physician often prescribes medication for already sensitive nerves.

Too often the cause, in the estimation of the patient and the physician, is of secondary importance; both patient and physician seek freedom from pain—or what causes it—in obliviousness rather than searching for the true source of the illness.

Even some so-called normal people shut themselves up inside their intellectual or emotional compartments and never think of keeping the other portions of their building in order. Under such conditions physicians often prescribe a change of climate, scenery and lifestyle, usually with unsatisfactory results; often exercise therapy can accomplish this goal. If one's general nutrition needs to be stimulated, exercise accomplishes this. If congestion is to be removed, exercise can accomplish this. If the level of peripheral circulation is to be raised, exercise therapy will provide the cure.

The system of movements provides selectivity over what function or force shall predominate in the individual. Several such organic actions may be those of nutrition, circulation, or waste and they can be awakened by movements in any parts of the body where they have become languid and insufficient.

It is worth noting that when symptoms of nervousness come on with acute paroxysms, they are frequently a result of visceral obstructions and derangements. An unhealthy change occurring suddenly in the contents of the alimentary canal may generate a peculiar product that poisons the blood or irritates the nerve centers of the body, sometimes producing severe and strange symptoms. These acute paroxysms generally subside spontaneously. The treatment through exercise should be directed to aiding the digestive powers, to raising the functional activity of the liver, and to restoring certain bodily secretions.

This therapy supplies the means for directly arousing the action of the nerves. In this way treatment can be offered to the stomach, liver, bowels, circulation of the head and feet, etc. When this is accomplished nervousness often will subside.

A careful reading of this book will enable the reader to prepare an exercise prescription suited for his own particular case.

Neurasthenia

This peculiar and distressing affliction indicates a diseased state of the nerves, rather than of the organ to which it is commonly associated. It may accompany that state of general nervousness described above; but sometimes those nerve centers that are situated in the lower section of the spinal cord, from which these organs draw their power, are the principal cause of the trouble. In either case there is a great amount of mental depression and lassitude accompanying this disease. The person so afflicted may be unable to enjoy life or even to take his proper place in society. Treatment must be general rather than topical, for topical treatment is often more harmful than helpful.

The best solution to this problem is to relieve nervous excitability. Some ways of accomplishing this have already been pointed out. Often the treatment required does not differ essentially from that required for neuralgia. General health must be restored before the symptoms disappear.

Neuralgia

This is a disease characterized by great pain, but it is usually unaccompanied by visible indications of inflammation, such as swelling, heat, and redness. Frequently there is even an absence of soreness. Hence it is presumed that the cause of the pain is confined to the nervous structure itself, and is not attributable to any unhealthy condition of the vital structures to which the painful nerve is distributed. Neuralgia may attack any portion of the body, whether internal or external. It may be confined to a particular locality, or it may affect the entire nervous system.

To understand this affliction it is necessary to inquire into the nature and causes of pain. The sensation of pain is the means by which the nervous system communicates to the mind that there is an activity occurring which is incompatible with the normal and healthy functioning of the body as a whole. However the pain of neuralgia seldom yields to ordinary medicinal influences, generally directed at masking the symptoms. These may temporarily obliterate the consciousness of pain. But the pain returns when the effects of the medication wear off.

It is wrong to expect that the disease will vanish while the nutritive processes carry on in an imperfect way. The body must be relieved of used up matter. Arterial blood, rich in oxygen, must again find its way to circulate freely to every structure before any permanent benefit can be experienced.

How exercise therapy can effect the removal of neuralgic pain is obvious. The amount of force exerted by a muscle corresponds to the amount of change that takes place in that muscle during its action. Pain, however severe, is the result of nerve-action, and consequently of nutritive change in the inner tissue of the nerve itself. If the nerve is diseased or has undergone such a drastic structural change that it is unable to perform its function, one is no longer conscious of pain in that part of the body.

Restoring afflicted nerves to health depends upon depressing their over-activity. In direct proportion to the increase in nervous activity is a decrease in muscular nutrition. The limb afflicted with sciatica becomes weak; the neuralgic subject has little muscular power. Thus, the nutritive effort is concentrated upon these over-excited nerves. Malnutrition of the nervous system is an important contributing factor in neuralgia—as is effectively proven by the immediate decrease in neuralgic pain when the activity of contiguous muscles is increased through exercises. The most important responsibility of the exercise cure is the perfection of the nutritive operations. To accomplish this, physical exercise is entirely sufficient. In this way, the outlets of the body are stimulated, and waste matters are eliminated; those matters necessary from the alimentary canal to maintain nutrition are selected and conveyed by the blood to their various points of destination. This is particularly the case with the saline elements of the blood, without which the organizing processes cannot take place.

The most painful cases of neuralgia are those attributed to mineral poisoning, which occurs with various trades, such as those working with gold, mercury, or other metals or their salts. The use of mineral drugs as a medicine is another source of this affliction. Many people who have suffered mineral poisoning are forever after subject to attacks of neuralgia. Physical exercise may be the only way of dislodging and conveying foreign matter such as this from the system. but even this is not always successful.

The prescription for neuralgia should take into account every part of the body affecting the purifying and blood-making processes which in their turn influence that part of the body subject to pain. Nutrition, and passive physical therapy such as stroking, clapping, punching, etc., as the case may require, are important elements. The single movements should consist of the passive portion applied to regions of the body that can be reached. When the neuralgic disorder is local, movements should be chosen that will act upon the muscles of that afflicted part, especially those near the origin of the pain.

9   Principles of Holistic Exercise Therapy

Physical culture for hygienic and medical purposes is by no means a new thing. Physical movement has been encouraged throughout every age. Its use may have been suggested by the natural instincts of the mind and its subsequent imperfect use has been pointed out through experience. Among Indian and African tribes, various manipulations and flagellations have been practiced, generally connected with tribal rituals, incantations, prayers, etc. It is well known that certain bodily movements produce vertigo, nausea, palpitations of the heart and various other symptoms similar to those brought on by chemical means. In the past people, who knew nothing of brain fatigue or of the confinement and ineffectual exercises connected with indoor and sedentary occupations, had no physical training other than the chase and the dance to which they were devoted. As it happened, their system of regulating health and overcoming disease developed naturally by the employment of physical exercise. But the system has been almost abandoned in today's world. Physical culture is not the attempt to

achieve athletic prowess, it is the attempt to condition
the body and maintain it in good health.

Physical exercise is receiving much superficial attention at the moment. Most of this attention is concerned
with pumping iron, jogging, and exercise designed for
flattening the stomach, popular subjects for authors.
Unfortunately, few practical precepts or definite directions are given.

The feeble person, the overweight person and the
invalid are constantly advised to exercise. Lecturers,
books, friends, and physicians all unite in this advice,
but none of them offers definite and satisfactory infor-
mation on how such people can attempt exercise and
how it should be applied. The individuals who can best
make use of the exercises described in this treatise are
those who engage in a prescriptive exercise program. In
such a program they have the opportunity to observe
their instructor or others in the program.

Unfortunately, many people are unable to locate qual-
ified instructors and thus are obliged to work on their
own.

In every community there is a large group of persons
who might be called partial-invalids—persons who don't
possess good health, but at the same time don't feel the
need of medical care. These people are aware of impending disease and can avoid it by holistic measures.
Current medical practice is cognizant of preventive medicine but doesn't do much about it except to confirm the
forewarning. Invalids are aware of this and so many keep
aloof from medical advice that insists upon their habitually taking drugs. Many times they can, if they know

how, press their various latent powers into activity and harmony, and many can soon achieve better health while pharmaceutical remedies would eventually cause their problems to worsen.

Another group of people who could benefit from this therapy are those whose avocations are sedentary, but every now and then require the continued and strenuous use of a large part of their muscles. These include many weekend athletes such as skiers, whose activities tend to place detrimental strain on many parts of the body. Their avocations are a potent cause of ill health. However, such ill effects can easily be counteracted through physical and nutritive therapy.

Generally, people who are engaged in sedentary work need physical and nutritive therapy to prevent them from falling into ill health. These people direct all the available forces of their body through a particular channel—the brain and nerves. This is contrary to the laws of their system, and so ill consequences usually follow. One set of functions is being heightened to the detriment of other sets of functions, which are becoming reduced in power and, in the end, are literally starved out. These people can, if they choose, learn how to counteract the disproportionate nervous wear and cultivate and maintain their physical vigor.

Physical culture, not a sports program, should be an integral part of every educational program, for the physical health of the average student is sadly neglected and students graduate physically uneducated. While sitting in the classroom listening to their teachers many students work hard intellectually but they also develop a lifelong lease on a narrow chest, shriveled and flabby muscles and a general dyspeptic habit.

The case seems worse with women. Usually they have even fewer opportunities for bodily activity than do men. Many prevalent diseases among older women are acquired because they have followed the customs of society and the neglect of physical culture. In this way women in their sixties and seventies acquire chlorosis, nervousness, dyspepsia, and deformities of the spine and chest, while younger women are afflicted with menstrual difficulties, infertility, and anemia.

The principle of cultivating the body along with the mind, so as to preserve health and emphasize mental culture is not new. It has been recognized and put into practice in ancient and modern times. But, in the United States we are just beginning to recognize the need for such holistic lifestyles.

10   Holistic Movement Principles

It is necessary to bear in mind the distinction between movements, gymnastics and exercises as these words are used in this book. Exercise is understood to mean all voluntary motions of the body, without any reference to the object or objects in view. Thus labor and recreation, practiced by either body or mind, whether general or partial, are exercise.

The word gymnastics is used exclusively to indicate the means of developing the corporeal frame for a special purpose, by certain exercises, Gymnastics are employed by those in good health, and are recognized universally as a useful means of developing the healthy body into its proper proportions which, without exercise, it fails to do.

The term exercises, however, does not include all that is implied in movements. Movements are not limited to muscular action initiated by the will, but include other motions as well, employed according to certain rules for specific, rational purposes. Movements, in short, are simply motions of specific kinds, having specific effects, practiced for specific purposes, and intended to secure definite results. Movements are mechanical agencies, directed upon either the whole system or a part of it, for the purpose of inducing determinate effects upon its vital actions.

Hence, the kind of movements proper in a given case are determined by the condition of the system, and will change with its variations so as to correspond with its special as well as general needs at the particular time when they are employed.

Types of Movements

Active and Passive. The division of movements into active and passive relates to the sources from which the moving power is derived. The motion of riding, for instance, is passive if the body is supported. So are clappings, knockings, kneadings, pullings, shakings, vibratings, etc., of the duplicated movements (see below), because both the motion and the will that give it energy are derived from another person.

Among the single movements there are none that is wholly passive. While the muscles of one portion of the body are acting upon other portions and the former are active and the latter passive. The condition of the will is an important element in determining whether the movement be active or passive.

Whenever the contractile power of a muscle is engaged in overcoming resistance, the resulting movement is active, or not whether the effort proves successful.

Single and Duplicated Movements. A movement is

called single when but a single person is engaged in its execution, duplicated when more than one is engaged. In single movements the weight of the whole body or some portion of the body is overcome by muscular action—as when in a standing position a leg or arm is raised. The movement is also single if the resistance of antagonizing muscles is overcome—as in twisting a limb or the trunk, or when a burden is added to the weight of the body, or to the extremity or part moved. The movements described in this book are single movements. But as frequent reference is made to duplicated movements, it is necessary to describe their general qualities and purposes.

Duplicated movements are of two kinds. In one, the movement is received by the patient, who is quite passive, while motion of some kind is given to some portion of the body, or to the whole of it. In the other kind, the patient is required to bring into action some particular part designated in the prescription—the quality, amount, and duration of the action is controlled by the physician. This action is varied according to the therapeutic indications of the case, partly as diagnosed by the physical symptoms observed, and partly as determined by the trained perception and experience of the operator. Through manipulation the operator offers a certain degree of resistance which aids in effecting the desired physiological action of the part concerned. The resistance should be carefully varied in the different stages, and should employ all the nuances of manipulation that are required in giving expression to a musical performance.

The range and variety of effects capable of being directed by duplicated movements are great, meeting most of the indications of chronic disease. These effects may be realized either in interior organs or the extremities, and they may be confined mainly to a particular anatomical area or physiological function—such as the nerves or muscles—or may influence all such elements together. These movements are adaptable to the most weakened invalid or to the heartiest persons, and never need produce effects beyond the requirements.

A most important element in the treatment by duplicated movements is that of cooperation, by both the will and action, of the patient with the physican or operator. Through such cooperation the superior power of one becomes a source of strength to the other.

Nothing so encourages a person as the consciousness of abundant ability, and this is fully supplied to the mind by the auxilliary power.

Consequently, in addition to the control obtained over the chemical and vito-chemical actions, one becomes able to secure the favorable influence of the healthy functioning of the nerves, thus restoring normal organic operations.

Single movements, on the other hand, being comparatively few in number and simple in character, are much more readily learned and practiced and have been found effective in combating the less critical forms of disease, thus preventing a more serious illness.

Concentric and Eccentric Movements. When the maximum output of the muscles is approximated, with muscular contraction steadily increasing, the movement is said to be concentric. When the muscle is stretched and its contraction is steadily decreasing, the movement is said to be eccentric. Thus, the raising of a book by one's hand, requires a concentric movement, while lowering the book gradually would require an eccentric movement. In both cases the same muscles have been employed. But often the effect upon circulation, and especially upon the innervation of the part, is entirely different. The advantages of this distinction are, however, only imperfectly available in the single movements, because both the concentric and eccentric movements are used indiscriminately in many of them. In practicing duplicated movements, it is easy to render a given movement either wholly concentric or eccentric so as to gain whatever advantages may be derived from this distinction.

To accomplish, for instance, an elbow bend via single-type movement, it is necessary for the muscles of the upper arm—toward which the forearm is drawn in the action—to contract. This mass of muscles is shown at a–b in figure 1. This is concentric action. But the muscles of the opposite side of the arm are by no means passive. If they were, the bending would be accomplished with a sudden jerk; this is prevented by the contraction of the opposing muscles. However this contraction in not sufficient to prevent the shortening of a–b, and the consequent motion of the forearm. At the same time the muscular mass, c–d, is steadily extended in opposition to its efforts. Its movement is called eccentric.

If while the muscle c–d is contracting and resistance is applied at the hand, then a–b will not contract during the movement, for its opposing force is already supplied by the resistance from without, and though drawn out, it remains relaxed during the movement. The effect of the movement is experienced in the contracting part.

Again, if force is applied to the hand, and a–b is drawn out as a result of that force, then the muscle c–d will not contract, and it will possess neither the physiological nor mechanical conditions for propelling forward the venous blood, but will remain entirely inactive. The only result of the movement will be the contraction of a–b, with the resulting influx of arterial blood. Futhermore, if the movement is made with resistance both ways, from 1–2 and from 2–1, the contraction would be first concentric in c–d and a–b, without any eccentric action. But if force is used to move the limb in the directions specified, while the muscles oppose the force which overcomes them, then both actions are eccentric, and there are no concentric actions. The understanding of these principles is of primary importance in the application of movements for the elimination of disease.

The pressure resulting from the contraction of a–b forces the arm's blood into the venous capillaries, while the drawing out of the muscles c–d extends the arteries, relieves them of pressure, and admits more arterial blood into the capillaries than before. In both cases the conditions are supplied for a new contraction: in one case, by excluding waste matter, and in the other by bringing fresh arterial blood to the acting organ.

General and Localized Movements. One of the most potent causes of disease is the habitual employment of the powers of the system in a partial or inharmonious manner. A person who constantly uses his brain to the neglect of his whole body, his senses rather than his muscles, his hands and arms in preference to his legs, or his legs instead of his abdominal muscles, cannot enjoy good health. In these cases nutrition progresses inordinately in the active parts, while other equally important but inactive parts of the body are suffering for want of nutrition. The effect after a time— and in invalids that period is soon reached—is a total collapse of the body's physical energies.

These instances illustrate a principle that is apt to be ignored by individuals and neglected by physicians. The moderate use of a part of the body while other parts are in a state of inactivity not only stimulates the nutrient actions in the excercised parts, but also causes the general current of the circulation to set in toward them to an abnormal extent. In other words, an excessive and continued use of an organ induces a tendency toward congestion of its tissues. It also generally heightens its nervous sensibility, frequently carrying it to the point of irritability. if an organ is set vigorously at work while all other parts are at rest, it is made to use the whole available vital force of the system. Any organ may be compelled to do this, and they may all be compelled in succession by sufficient stimulation. If the organs of the body are employed in union or in proper succession, the current of the circulation is thus set in motion in them. Instead of producing congestion and irritation, it then provides the proper conditions for the high degree of nutrition necessary for their long and continued use. At the same time it prevents the healthful functioning of other parts, so that those most vascular and delicate organs are injured.

The state of congestion and the opposite state of shrunken capillaries coexist in different parts of the body in nearly all cases of chronic disease. The capillaries of some portions are distended and too weak to push forward their contents, and the stagnant blood deteriorates and becomes incapable of affording nutrition. At the same time other capillaries, generally those of the skin and extremities, do not receive enough blood to meet their nutritional needs. The rate of the circulation is unequal, since the blood is arrested in the congested organ. The final cause of such trouble may be a poor quality of blood, but behind this there remain causes connected with the blood-making processes of the body, which properly applied movements are capable of correcting.

The removal of congestion is one of the primary objectives of partial movements. A congested organ is one in which the capillaries have lost their contractability, and are therefore distended with blood. Most of the local, passive duplicated movements assist in the efforts to remove this condition. But permanent effects are secured by arousing vital action in—and consequently drawing the congested fluid to—contiguous organs, and even organs remote from the seat of disease. Thus the afflicted part is emptied and relieved, and consequently acquires a healthy tone in its capillary circulation, as do other organs that were suffering from deficient nutrition. If good judgment is employed in the selection and arrangement of the movements in the prescription, no more efficient means can be found for relieving congestion.

A similiar principle is concerned in the treatment of disordered innervation. If a single organ is the chief medium of nervous action, or even if it be the seat of great pain, other organs are proportionately wanting in sensibility. Nervous power is dependent upon the general conditions of nutritive supply or muscular power. Congestion and poor innervation may be removed from any locality by employing movements in other portions of the system.

The attempts to accomplish these objectives through ordinary medical means are less successful than through movements because the control of the circulation thus obtained is less direct and perfect. These principles furnish suggestions for the management of the sick. They provide a means of reversing those mysterious and subtle operations of the system whereby diseases are originally produced. And these principles are capable of easy and satisfactory demonstration.

The curative employment of movements is by no means confined to local applications. Those involving the whole body are often used to excellent advantage. Such movements urge the blood into the capillaries and increase the peripheral circulation. But they need to be employed with much discretion in order to avoid fatigue and the subsequent failure of the purpose for which they are supplied.

The Use of Movements

Influence of Movements. It is already understood that the muscles and nerves are two great channels through which the available powers of the human system are made to work.

In health, the muscles and nerves exercise coordinated functions. The muscles act only in response to nervous stimuli, and this involves both mental and sensorial actions, for the origin of the impulses imparted to the muscles resides in the intellect and sensorium. The voluntary muscles ordinarily obey only the mandates of the will and feelings.

Disease, arising from whatever cause, involves a disturbance in the operation of these two classes of powers. Muscular power is partially or wholly suspended, while the sensorial power is generally increased, frequently to the point of pain. If the proper relationship between these two sets of powers is habitually disregarded, disease in some form will be the inevitable consequence.

The chronic invalid is tormented with sensations, and often with those that seem to bear slight relationship to his apparent disease. In these cases the imagination is stimulated to excess; the strongest wish of such an individual is incapable of resisting the powers of feelings and fancies that exaggerate with the progression of his illness.

Much of the disease of our modern civilization has its origins in this partial function, which in turn produces partial development—which is another name for deformity. The nervous system is, in many cases, compelled to act constantly—and with a force greatly disproportionate to the musclar system.

If the body's constitution is defective from hereditary causes, its tendency toward disease of this kind is proportionately stronger, and the necessity for intelligent training of the system's nerve-power becomes even more imperative. If such a nervous habit is prolonged and the muscles continue to be deprived of their nutrition, the general nutrient actions throughout the body will be weakened.

Abuse of the nervous system usually operates through two channels: the mental and the sensorial. Examples of the latter are much more numerous than those of the former, but those of a mental nature often occur in conjunction with those of a sensorial nature. The sensorial faculties minister to the material welfare and gratification of the body. But whenever the nerves belonging to this class are inordinately stimulated—that is, when stimulated without reference to nutritive ends—they become overstrained. The nutrition of the parts is perverted, their powers debilitated, and their action uncontrollable.

When the emotions have undue influence they operate in a similarly injurious way. The excitements of extensive or precarious business or of marital discord also produce these effects. Feelings sometimes arouse disastrous physiological conditions.

In all cases, arising from whatever cause, the use of movements furnishes a direct, safe, powerful and philosophical means of restoring interrupted harmonies and correcting ill health, provided the influence of the causes leading to illness is withdrawn.

The Will and the Muscles in Movements. Most people seem to think that the degree of fatigue one experiences indicates the amount of exercise performed but it really only shows the amount of energy put forth, which depends upon the will. The degree of fatigue and the amount of exercise do not necessarily bear a direct relationship to each other. As evidence that fatigue is connected with the exercise of the will, it is only necessary to refer to numerous physiological operations that proceed without our attention and without fatigue. Some are capable of being brought into relationship with the will, and thereby immediately become fatiguing. The heart's action, though powerful and incessant, is unaccompanied by any sense of fatigue. The internal organs, such as the stomach and intestinal tract, are in constant motion, but never grow weary. The motion of riding in a train or automobile is not fatiguing. Many of the ordinary avocations of life are habitual, and are performed automatically and without fatigue. In these movements the will is inactive; such actions are often under the control of the involuntary or cerebro-spinal system of nerves.

The function of respiration affords an excellent illustration of the relationship between the will and the involuntary nerves in movements. In ordinary respiration there is no fatigue because it proceeds without consciousness; that is, it is involuntary. But when we control this function through use of the will, its performance is immediately followed by exhaustion.

A careful analysis leads us to the principle that the amount of direct fatigue experienced is in direct proportion to the amount of mental and nervous energy exerted, not the amount of muscular action employed. And this proportion seems to be determined chiefly by the amount of time required in executing the movements, the quick movements requiring the greatest expenditure of nervous power. The principle here is that velocity is obtained at the expense of power.

If the movement is slower, the amount of muscular action is greater in proportion to the time required. This principle is made evident by the physiology of muscular contraction, where the longer the action of the muscle is continued, the greater the number of its ultimate elements that participate in the action.

Rapid movements necessitate the most nervous action; slow and sustained movements, the most muscular action. If the principle is stated with reference to the limits of these powers, it might be said that the one exhausts the most nervous, and the other the most muscular power. In terms of nutrition, the one stimulates the most nervous, and the other the most muscular power.

This principle is well illustrated in common experience. If a person runs a few feet briskly, he will pant with fatigue; if he walks the same distance, he is refreshed and invigorated. However, the total amount of mechanical resistance that he has overcome is greater in the latter case than in the former. In the first instance the objective was accomplished by means of a greater effort than in the second; but in the second, a larger number of muscle cells had taken part in the contraction than in the first. In the one case a larger amount of blood was conveyed to the nerve centers to sustain the action; in the other case, the muscles received the larger quantity of blood to replenish the waste resulting from their action.

This principle finds firm substantiation in all departments of pathology. The paralytic walks with great difficulty because, though the muscles are really unaffected, the will is transmitted to them imperfectly and through great effort because of the debilitated state of the nerve conductors.

The effect of poisons upon the nervous system presents a pathological state supporting this principle. Strychnine produces violent muscular contortion, exhibiting evidence of the excited and rapid action—and finally the exhaustion—of the nerve centers. Spirits and most other stimulants produce their deceptive effect by exciting in the nerve-centers an action which the deluded victim attempts to maintain by repeating the doses. No lasting power is really gained in any of these ways, because the action is essentially destructive, not constructive.

In the movement cure, these general principles are directly applied, hence its therapeutic value. It employs slow movements in preference to the more rapid, because invalids need to have their nervous powers conserved, and their general muscular and nutritive powers increased. Such invalids have suffered enough from unnatural and irregular nervous activity. The muscles of such patients not only fail to respond, but also fail to control properly the productive actions that directly depend upon a full supply of nervous energy in the muscular system. We need to be careful that our practice in making remedial application of movements corresponds with these principles. Not only application of the movements, but also the general habits of the body, must be made to agree with the same principles.

Movements as Therapy. The single movements approximate the duplicated movements in importance as a therapeutic means. The latter answer all the distinct purposes indicated in chronic disease. Their effects may

be localized as well as general, and in this respect their
therapeutic results equal those of drugs, difficult as some
may find it to believe. The primary impression made by
a drug is essentially pathological; while that of a movement is in the direction of the desired physiological action, and consequently of good health. Movements are
also superior to drugs in the extent to which the physiological actions may be influenced by them, especially
in the control over the circulation of the blood, and the
directness with which respiration and nutrition are influenced. Such results can hardly be expected under the
administration of drugs.

The outstanding difference between movements and
drugs can be found in their respective relationships to
the system. The one changes physiological action to path-
logical, the other carries pathological action toward physiological. The drug accomplishes specific objectives by
pervading the entire organism, leaving a weakened condition. It has no power to stimulate the life force of the
system. Movements, on the other hand, secure or restore
unity and balance to the various functions.

Movements as a Source of Nutritive Medication. Much
is said in regard to supplying the blood with its saline
ingredients. It so happens that ordinary food furnishes
an abundance of usable nutritive matters. The trouble
is not in the lack of such material, but the power to make
use of it. The question is, are the bodily structures in
a state of readiness and fitness to receive and appropriate
the supplies? It is contrary to physiological law to conclude that nutritive actions can proceed effectively in the
absence of the conditions necessary for the supply of
oxygen.

If we chemically test any proper and wholesome foods we shall find saline and other matters present in quantities positively above the demands of the system. These matters are constituents of all common food. Whether they are utilized or are cast off depends entirely upon the needs of the organism and its appropriating ability. This need exists in direct, uniform ratio to the waste; and though the blood and tissues might be deficient in these substances, they can never become richer in them in the absence of imperative and effectual demand created by action. Movements provide the means for bringing nutritive materials and the saline elements of the blood from the cavity of the stomach into the inner chambers of the system, where they are needed.

The saline elements of food are in a state of preparation as effected by plants expressly for nutritive purposes. Iron, lime, phosphorous, etc., are not in food as crude substances, but are incorporated with other elements in organic combination, thus suitable to proceed to every needy tissue of the body.

Movements Vs. Nerve Stimulants. Few people fully understand the impropriety, from a physiological point of view, of subjecting their nerves to the habitual influence of sedatives and stimulants. These agents contribute to what is technically termed retrograde metamorphosis in the body. Such chemicals debase the system and interfere with nature's design for the production of normal physiological changes in the system. Movements offer a ready way of quieting the nerves by the simplest of means. Distressful sensations sometimes indicate that dead matter needs to be ejected from the system, and the most effectual way of accomplishing such removal is through movements.

Movements and Pathology. The understanding of pathology changes when seen from the point of view furnished by movements. The cure of disease is no longer solely the province of unintelligible operations or mysterious mixtures. Pain need no longer be confused with disease, nor is the cure completed when the consciousness has become oblivious to suffering.

On the contrary, disease depends on disturbed physiological action, and it waits only for correct and consistent action to be restored. The special conditions upon which the symptoms of disease are based are easily and speedily removable when they exist in moderate degree.

Several of these removable causes or conditions usually co-exist in the same case, but with different degrees of intensity or development. Movement seeks to recover the impaired harmony of the system and never, like drugs, develops symptoms of its own worse than the disease. By bringing all the forces of the organism into due co-relation, movement assists the system to glide naturally back to health.

These invisible, vito-chemical actions are capable of producing visible physiological results. We are not accomplishing much when we apply antidotes to effects, while the causes are busily at work out of sight and out of reach.

The inter-relationships of physiological and pathological agencies are so involved that to look for the initial cause of disease is like seeking the end of a circle, or a needle in a hay stack. The essential phenomena are recognizable; defective respiration, congestion or mal-circulation, imperfect nutrition, and poor innervation. These are the conditions that chiefly interest us, and those which we seek to control.

Function of Movements. Whether movements are hygienic or remedial in their effects depends upon the character of the case for which they are used. They are hygienic when their influences maintain the already-existing healthy relationships of the physiological man—when they give a healthy scope to all vital powers, in spite of the deteriorating tendencies brought on by sedentary lifestyles.

Movements thus applied may be called the natural means of counteracting the evil tendencies of an artificial mode of life.

Movements become medical in nature when their effects are to improve imperfect physiological relations, or break up pathological states habitually existing; as, for instance, when they permanently increase the circulation and nutrition of a part previously defective, increase the respiration, or diminish poor innervation, restrain unhealthy discharges, or restore any defective functions to a healthful and satisfactory state.

Movements and Morale. Invalids gain instruction through their experience in the daily use of movements in regard to the causes of their troubles, and thus can rise above the depressing influence of disease. Through movements the invalid no longer pursues remedies for difficulties that he is continually reproducing in himself.

11 Applying Holistic Movements.

The physical movement treatment regards the system as subject to a continual though invisible growth, and to further and perfect this process is its special aim and business. As the pulling-down and repairing operations of the system in health are gradually and unconsciously conducted, so too are the favorable effects of judicious treatment being imperceptibly produced. The patient realizes the effects of this treatment only by experiencing decrease in his pains and a restoration of strength and vivacity.

Scheduling of Treatment. If the purpose is to counteract the effects of sedentary habits, of undue mental application or physical overexertion, movements may be taken at any time. In cases of disease, it is desirable that they be taken in the early part of the day when, owing to the previous night's rest, there is more energy.

In general, movements should be practiced no more than once a day. And however moderately used, we must guard against the possible crises, such as headaches, febrile symptoms, etc., which may occur after a short term of treatment. Upon the occurrence of such symptoms, we must immediately change the prescription or temporarily discontinue treatment altogether, for the effects in such cases are similiar to those brought about by the abuse of drugs.

An auxiliary prescription may sometimes be made for another time in the day, repeating perhaps some portion of the original one, but this should only be done under the direction of a competent physician.

Manner of Treatment. Every movement has two important elements—mechanical and mental—neither of which may be neglected for the other. Correct posture must be assumed. The part to be moved should be made to pass through the prescribed line until it reaches the indicated limit, which is usually the limit of the contractile capacity of the chief muscles employed; the last position should then be maintained for a few minutes. Finally, the part in motion is returned to its original position with comparatively little muscular effort.

In the meantime, the mind or will is intent on the mechanical execution of the movement, and the nerves are busy conveying the necessary stimuli to the part, without which the execution of the movement, if it is a voluntary one, is impossible. The mind is engaged in sustaining the vital operations of the moving part. Both the external display of mechanical force, and the internal vito-chemical changes upon which it depends, are the results of mental action. If the prescription lacks precision, intelligent determination and force, little is accomplished.

Rhythm. This element of the treatment is highly important, and one that must not be overlooked. The physical movements should be performed slowly, much more slowly than are the habitual motions of the body. Thus the acting part occupies the attention for a considerable time, and the amount of control gained over the changes of the part is consequently and proportionately great, while the energy of the will and the expenditure of nerve-power that is required is small. The absolute time occupied in a movement should vary with the size, and particularly the length, of the acting muscle or muscles, the shorter muscles doing their work in shorter time spans. The part should then retain its extreme position for a short period.

Exertion. In duplicated movements the assistant is totally in control of the amount of exertion employed by the patient. The effect may be perfectly graduated to suit his judgment.

The single movements do not offer this type of precise control. The resistance is supplied by the weight of the part which is varied as the positions vary, and can be increased only to a limited extent. The amount of exertion possible in any position is dependent upon the degree of mobility of the part concerned.

Number. The number of movements to be taken at one time should be sufficient enough to engage all parts of the system (there are some exceptions to this rule—cases of paralysis and surgical diseases), but not so much as to develop fatigue, or only such moderate fatigue as is quickly recovered from. The number generally required ranges from ten to twelve.

Order. This is a very important matter in duplicated movements: so much so that a re-arrangement of the order may produce different effects. The arrangement should be such that the movements support each other and work together to produce the desired effect. An intense arrangement would cause them to interfere with and neutralize each other.

A proper arrangement is also important in the single movements. Too many applied in succession to the same organ, if diseased, would be likely to produce congestion. The usual effect of excessive exercise, if the part is diseased, would tend to increase and accelerate the disease. All requirements of the system, in any given case, should be considered in the prescription. It is suggested that the following order be individually adapted to meet the needs of each particular case:

1. A respiratory movement.
2. A movement of the lower extremities.
3. A movement of the upper extremities.
4. A movement of the abdomen.
5. A movement of the lower extremities.
6. A respiratory movement to finish.

Whatever the order, the movements should always harmonize with each other. For it is only from the harmonious union of their separate actions that the best results can be achieved.

Relation to Diseased Parts. Every formula of movements for persons who have a local weakness or disease will contain both general and special elements—the latter having particular reference to the disease. But, active movements must not be applied to organs affected with actual disease. The diseased part must be approached gradually. beginning at some remote part of the body, slowly arousing it to vital activity, and augmenting its capacity to receive blood. In this way congestion accompanying the disease is gradually removed, and the vital and nutrient power of the system is increased and established, until finally the diseased part is so relieved that it becomes capable of advantageously receiving the direct effects of movement.

The passive kind of duplicated movements are, however, an exception. The direct effect of such passive movements as vibrations is to move the blood from the congested capillaries toward the veins. The adherent corpuscles are thus dislodged and the blood flow arrested by them is allowed to move onward. Such movements greatly assist in the removal of congestion and may, with care, be applied to the diseased members or organs.

The general habits of exercise should be in accord with the movement prescription. For instance, as in proportion to the organic disturbances there is always an increase in nervous excitability and a decrease in physical power, the habitual exercises of the patient should be ordered to assist in repressing the excitability and to invigorate the general nutrition of the body. All violent and continued exercises that exhaust the powers and induce lasting fatigue should be avoided. Those that are partly passive, such as riding, sailing, travelling, etc., are highly appropiate, and may be taken with great benefit.

Regions of the Body. Movements necessarily have special relationships to the body's individual parts, or region, with no definite portion of its mass having distinct boundaries. The term is very general, and an area of the body thus designated includes a portion of the whole of several anatomical divisions. By thus simplifying the terminology, a knowledge of anatomy on the part of the assistant applying movements is dispensed with and the intelligent and successful use of single movements is made practicable.

A region generally consists of one or more joints, including the bones, ligaments, muscles, nerves, vessels, areolar tissues, and other elements of that organ within that locality. Each joint is considered a center of motions with the invisible physiological or nutritive actions permanently connected with the health of the part. If the impulse to motion proceeds from external sources then the region simply indicates the structures acted upon.

Any portion of the body, however complex in its structure and functions, which may be moved en masse and separately from the rest of the framework, constitutes a region. The whole trunk, or even a part of it may, if included in a movement, be thus considered.

This system is different from the drug system which is primarily applied to the stomach and alimentary canal, while that portion of it which is received into the circulation subsequently spends its power among the vital structures, generally and indiscriminately, wherever the blood circulates, in the healthy as well as diseased portions.

In the application of the movement cure, however, only those parts needing help are singled out in the prescription.

12   Terminology of Positions

Five principal positions are used in the movements: standing, kneeling, sitting, lying, and hanging.

Each of these positions has several variations.

THE TRUNK

I. Standing Positions

1. ERECT-STANDING—In this important position the body is upright and vertical, the arms hanging by the sides, the legs parallel, the heels in contact, the toes about twelve inches apart.

2. FALL-STANDING—The whole body inclines at an angle from the perpendicular, all the members retaining their natural relative positions. The body in this position must be supported at some point by a firm object. A slight deviation forward is called inclining; backward, reclining.

The body may greatly deviate from the perpendicular,

and the position is then called low fall-standing; when it deviates slightly, it is called high fall-standing.

It may deviate in any direction—forward, right, left, or backward—and to various degrees in these directions. The position is described with sufficient accuracy by designating the cardinal positions between which the body falls as forward-sidewise, right or left, and backward-sidewise, right or left.

3. *BENT-STANDING*—This indicates that the trunk is bent at the center. Deep-bent means bent to the utmost extent. The bending may be either forward, sidewise, or backward, and to any degree.

II. Kneeling Positions

1. *ERECT-KNEELING*—In this position the weight of the trunk rests on the knees instead of the feet. A soft cushion must be placed under the knees.

2. *FALL-KNEELING*—Here the trunk may assume the falling position while kneeling, corresponding with the fall-standing position.

III. Sitting Positions

The variations of this position relate to the disposition of the legs as well as of the trunk.

2. *SITTING*—The trunk rests upon the buttocks, the thighs at right angles to the body at the hips and to the lower legs at the knees, the feet resting upon the floor.

2. SHORT-SITTING—The buttocks rest upon the edge of the chair, occupying as little of it as is possible while maintaining proper posture.

3. LONG-SITTING—The legs are extended horizontally in the same plane with the buttocks, while the trunk is erect.

4. LIE-SITTING, or HALF-LYING—In this position the trunk reclines, and is supported by cushions or a movable seat constructed for this purpose.

5. FALL-SITTING—The trunk deviates from the perpendicular at a certain angle, greater or less; thus it may be falling, inclining, or deep-falling.

Fall-sitting may also be forward, sidewise, backward, or on any intermediate point.

6. STRIDE-SITTING—This indicates that the legs are placed apart at right angles, and also that the feet are widely separated, so as to afford as broad a base as possible.

IV. Lying Positions

In these positions the whole body is horizontal. These positions are to be varied by changing the points of support.

1. FORWARD-FALL—In this position the face is down, the body extended on a cushion.

2. BACKWARD-LYING—Here the face is up, the body extended upon the back.

3. SIDEWISE-LYING—Body extended upon the right or left side.

4. *TRUNK-LYING*—In this position only the trunk is supported, while the legs project beyond the supporting surface, and are sustained by the muscles. The variations are:

  a. Trunk-forward lying,
  b. Trunk-backward-lying, and
  c. Trunk-sidewise-lying.

5. *LEG-LYING*—In this position only the legs rest upon a suitable couch or seat while the trunk projects, sustained only by the action of the muscles. It affords the same variations as trunk-lying.

In leg-lying it is always necessary to employ some weight on the legs for balance.

This position offers the same modifications as trunk-lying.

6. *HEAD-AND-HEELS-LYING*—In this position the head and heels are supported by cushioned stools, while the body is extended horizontally between them, back down, sustained by the muscles.

7. *ELBOWS-AND-TOES-LYING*—In this position the body is supported only by the elbows and toes.

8. *SIDEWISE-LYING*—This affords several variations. Plain, elbow and foot, right, left, etc.

9. *BALANCE-LYING*—In this position the support for the body is under the center of the trunk. The position may also be backward, forward, or sidewise.

V.Hanging Positions

In this position the body is perpendicular and its weight is taken by the hands grasping an overhead pole.

SWIM-HANGING. Here the body is made to deviate from the perpendicular position with the assistance of another person.

THE ARMS

In each of the above postures of the body, the arms and legs may assume all the various positions that are consistent with the anatomical arrangement of the parts concerned. These variations of position are dependent upon the nature of the joints which connect these extremities with the trunk.

The joints of the ball-and-socket kind permit the greatest degree of freedom and motion. The arms are capable of rotating in an entire circle, of which the shoulder is the center.

In Figure 2, the arm positions are represented in the plane of the transverse diameter of the body. The left side of the body in the figure represents the chief positions of the arms in that plane. A is a shoulder joint, the center of the circle of which the arm is the radius. The names of these positions are as follows:

STRETCH, or *UPWARD-STRETCH: Aa*.

SIDE-STRETCH, or *YARD: Ac*.

HIGH-SIDE-STRETCH, or *LOW-YARD: Ad*.

DOWNWARD-STRETCH, or *NATURAL POSITION: Ae*.

The right side of the body in the figure represents the same positions but with the elbow bent at a right angle. A is again the shoulder joint.

Each of these positions receives the same name as the corresponding ones of the opposite side, with the addition of the term *Elbow-Bent*, to denote the deviation of the forearm from a straight line with the upper arm.

The following terms are used to denote specific arm positions in figure 2:

CURVE—A l o, indicates that the elbow and wrist joints are bent so as to bring the whole arm in close contact with the head. This is otherwise expressed as stretch, elbow, and wrist-bent rest.

SHELTER—A m l, is equivalent to high side-stretch, or yard, elbow-bent rest.

HEAVE—A n k, is the same as yard elbow-bent.

ANGLE—A i j, is low-yard elbow upward-bent.

WING—A i h, is low-yard elbow downward-bent rest.

COVER—C g f, is down-stretch elbow-bent rest.

The above comprises all the arm positions in the transverse plane of the body. The same kinds and number of positions, with slight variations, may be employed in any other plane.

Side View

Figure 3 represents the positions of the arms in the plane corresponding with the front-to-back diameter of the body. Because the shoulder is the center, the arm may describe the greater part of the circle of which it is the radius, except for a small arc at the rear.

It should also be noted that when the arm is extended perpendicularly, either up or down, it is in exactly the same position it occupies on the plane of figure 2, with the plane in this figure at right angles. The positions of the arms shown in figure 3 are as follows:

RACK, or *FORWARD-STRETCH:* ab.
HIGH-RACK, or *HIGH FORWARD-STRETCH:* Aa.
LOW-RACK, or *LOW FORWARD-STRETCH:* Ac.
BACKWARD-STRETCH: Ad.

THE LEGS

The leg positions are produced by the bending of the hip and knee joints, except in standing, lying, etc., when the lower extremities are parallel with the trunk. The movement of the hip joint is not quite so great as that of the shoulder joint, since it is limited in its mobility upward, but in general the positions of the legs correspond with those previously described for the arms.

The general term given to any deviation of the leg from the perpendicular produced by bending the hip joint, is kick:

FORWARD-KICK—The leg is carried forward and raised to an angle of about forty-five degrees.

HIGH-FORWARD-KICK—Is between forward-kick and the horizontal.

LOW-FORWARD-KICK—Is between forward kick and the perpendicular.

SIDEWISE-KICK—The leg is extended sidewise.

BACKWARD-KICK—The leg is extended backward.

There are also intermediate positions such as:

FORWARD-SIDEWISE-KICK—High and low.

BACKWARD-SIDEWISE—High and low.

These positions are designated by the term *knee-bent* prefixed to the names of positions resulting from the flexing of the thigh joint.

A number of positions of the legs, as in the case of the arms, are better expressed by distinct terms, as follows:

1. STRIDE—In this position the legs are set apart about two-and-a-half-feet on each side of the perpendicular, whether sitting, standing, or lying.

2. WALK—One leg is placed before the other, the trunk perpendicular between them, as in ordinary walking.

3. STEP-STANDING—One foot rests upon a step or stool, eight to twelve inches high. The leg may be extended either forward or sidewise.

4. FOOT-SUPPORT-STANDING—When this term is used, the position of the leg must also be designated, a matter often neglected in step-standing. Thus, forward-kick, foot-support, half-standing, indicates that while the body rests upon one leg, the other is raised in forward-kick position, and that the foot rests upon some object that elevates it from the floor.

5. SQUAT-POSITION—Both thigh and knee are bent at right angles.

6. LEG-ANGLE—A term indicating the bending of both hip and knee, without denoting degree.

In describing positions, the word *half* denotes that only one side is concerned, whether in reference to the arms or legs.

13   Single Movements: The Feet

A large number of small bones comprise the feet, and are firmly bound together by numerous ligaments and tendons. Some of the muscles of this region are confined to the feet, while others extend beyond and are attached to the bones of the leg, some nearly as high as the knee. Motion of the feet is produced by the action of those muscles, most of which are situated in the lower leg. The feet are constructed so as to be very elastic while at the same time they are very compact and strong.

The strength of the muscles and tendons of the feet is subjected to more constant stress than that of almost any other portion of the body. This results from their location, which demands that they not only sustain the weight of the entire superior portion of the body, but also any additional weight that the body may carry. Thus, we brace ourselves with the feet in performing any action by means of the upper extremities—as in lifting a weight, pushing, pulling, etc.

To maintain the normal perpendicular position of the body upon the narrow base furnished by the feet requires a stronger action of the muscles of the lower extremities than of those on any other part of the body. In contrast, in other animals the weight is shared by four legs, which gives a base so broad as to render any such concentration of muscular power unnecessary.

At first this arrangement in the human framework may seem to be unfavorable, however there is a wise provision of nature in the compensation of balance. At one end of the body is the head, containing the human brain which distinguishes the thinking man from the unthinking beasts. The functions of this part of the body require much nutrition. Now, to maintain an equilibrium of the circulation, it is necessary that the inferior extremities of the body should be subject to habitual and vigorous action so as to make an equally great demand upon circulation.

Consequently, it seems that when the health suffers from excessive cerebral action, the true remedy is strong action of the lower part of the body, especially at the feet, to bring about an equilibrium of the circulation. And as the demand for nutrition in those regions is answered, the unhealthy cerebral symptoms will abate. This principle is practiced in the application of irritants to the feet, the effect is equally realized by exercise. The technical term for such an achieved effect is *derivative*.

Movements of the lower extremities supply a ready means of counteracting the effects of excessive stimulation to the superior portions of the body and of the mental labor and anxieties associated with modern living. They also provide an efficient means for treatment of many cases of chronic disease.

It is important to note that the feet are in close contact

with the earth, which is cooler and damper than the air which surrounds the rest of the body. Consequently, they lose heat more rapidly than do other portions of the body. To replenish this loss it is necessary to activate the heat-making process in the feet by forcing the blood to flow into these extremities. This can be achieved through the application of movements.

The reader must bear in mind that the following movements can only have curative or recuperative effects if they are practiced in conformity with the directions and principles laid down. To accomplish any good, they must be performed very slowly and with utmost precision.

1. Standing, Feet Extending

POSITION—Stand erect with one hand extended and touching a wall, chair, or other object.

ACTION—The feet should stretch at the ankle joint in such a way as to slowly raise the whole body as high as possible in tip-toe position, which must be sustained for a few minutes. Then relax the stretched muscles slowly until the heel reaches the floor and the feet and trunk have returned to their original position. This action should be repeated from six to ten times—slowly at first—with slight intervals between. If a more strenuous exercise of the muscles is desired, the movement may be performed with one foot only. After performing it with one foot, change to the other and repeat the movement in the same manner.

EFFECT—In this movement the muscles of the bot-

toms of the feet, as well as those of the posterior parts
of the legs below the knee, are brought into powerful
action, strengthened—that is, their nutrition is increased—due to the blood being attracted to the active
parts and away from the other organs. Hence, the term
derivative is applied to these actions.

2. Half-Standing, Heel-Pressing

POSITION—One foot is lifted behind the body, its
upper surface resting upon a cushioned seat or chair,
while the weight of the body is on the other leg, standing
in the erect position. The hand on the side of the raised
foot is placed upon it, requiring the body to be slightly
turned in that direction.

ACTION—First the hand is pressed upon the heel of
the foot, stretching the muscles and forcing the upper
surface of the foot into alignment with the leg, where it
remains for a short time. Next the ankle bends, raising
the heel against the pressure of the hand, until the foot
is at right angles with the leg. This action is to be repeated
six or eight times with each foot.

EFFECT—This movement makes the ankle supple,
warms the feet, and is powerfully derivative. The muscles of the top of the foot and sides of the lower leg are
chiefly affected.

3. Wing-Walk, Toe-Wall-Standing

POSITION—The hands should be placed upon the
hips, one foot advanced a yard or so beyond the other

in walking position, but with the ankle of the forward leg a good deal bent, and the toe against the wall, with the heel as near the wall as possible.

ACTION—First the knee of the forward leg should bend, causing the instep to form a more acute angle with the leg. This position is to be maintained for only a short time. Next the bent knee should be extended, and the ankle and foot made to resume their former position. figure 4 shows the posture, the dotted outline indicating the position at the end of the first part of the movement. This should be repeated five or six times with each foot.

EFFECT—The calf of the leg is strongly acted upon—as well as the sole of the foot—producing a derivative effect. This renders the ankle support supple, and the calf strong and elastic.

In each of the preceding movements the weight of the body is the chief resistance that the acting muscles are compelled to overcome.

4. Feet Sidewise Bending

POSITION—Sitting comfortably in a chair, the hands on the hips, the legs are extended horizontally across another chair that is placed immediately in front. The feet should extend beyond the supporting chair.

ACTION—First the feet should be slowly turned to one side, as far as they will go, while being held together. They should remain so for a short period. Next, they should be turned in in the opposite direction in the same manner. The action should be repeated ten or twelve times.

EFFECT—This motion is produced chiefly by the muscles of the lower leg and, in strengthening these parts, is derivative. If the ankle is weak so that it is inclined to bend too easily in one direction, the movement should be directed to that side. Slight deformities of the ankle may be corrected by persevering in this discipline of the faulty muscles.

5. Feet Rotation

POSITION—This is the same as in the preceding movement.

ACTION—The toes of both feet are made to describe as broad a circle as possible by slowly revolving clockwise ten or twelve times and then reversing the action. The motion is from the ankles and direction may be changed three or four times. The feet are to be kept close together during the execution of the movement, and the legs and body must remain in a uniform position.

EFFECT—In this movement all of the muscles of the feet and lower leg are put into vigorous action, and all the motions of which the ankle joint is capable are effected at each revolution. The movement is strongly derivative, and especially useful to the joint when in a weakened state.

6. Foot-Percussion (Passive)

POSITION—Begin by sitting in a chair with the lower part of one leg supported by the thigh of the other, the foot projecting a little beyond it, while the other foot rests firmly upon the floor.

ACTION—The hand on the side next to the raised foot holds a ruler or stick fifteen inches long and a half an inch thick, with which thirty or forty light blows are tapped upon the sole of the uplifted foot. The sole of the foot should be protected by a slipper. Both feet are to be acted upon alternately. This is called a passive movement because the effect derived is not produced by inducing muscular contractions of the part.

EFFECT—The benefit derived chiefly belongs to the capillaries and nerves of the part. The clogged vessels in the capillaries have their blood renewed while the arteries, through the increased action of the nerves supplying them, are made to contract more vigorously. If there is congestion of the capillaries—as in chilblains—it is quickly remedied, and the normal condition restored. The movement is derivative and warms the feet. The cure of chilblains by this method is speedy and permanent.

7. Foot-Rotation (Passive)

POSITION—This is the same as in the preceding movement, except that the hand, instead of holding a stick, grasps the toe of the foot.

ACTION—The toe of the held foot is made to describe as broad a circle as the ankle joint will allow, the foot itself remaining quite passive, offering no muscular resistance. The motion is wholly effected by means of the hand applied to it. The foot should make six revolutions in one direction, and then as many in the opposite. This change should be repeated five or six times and applied to both feet.

EFFECT—The foot may be turned farther in each direction in this manner than by its own muscles, and the movement is made with less effort and more pleasing effect.

8. Leg-Swinging

POSITION—Begin by standing with one foot on a stool. One hand is extended to touch a wall and provide balance while one leg hangs free.

ACTION—The free leg is forced to swing by bending at the hip joint, in a plane parallel with the front-to-back diameter of the body, the arc of a circle. Repeat this fifteen or twenty times on each side.

EFFECT—This motion assists the flow of the arterial blood toward the feet, while it retards the venous flow in the opposite direction, thereby causing the blood to accumulate in the lower extremities. This action warms the feet and induces a pleasant sensation in the limbs.

All the above movements, used regularly increase the healthful flow of arterial blood to the lower legs and feet and encouraging quck removal of the venous blood. They augment the bulk and energy of the active parts, warm the extremities, and bring relief to a system suffering from congestion or fatigue in its superior portions.

14   Single Movements: The Legs

The legs are endowed with very large masses of muscles, and it is necessary to employ them freely in movements in order to secure the objectives of our prescriptions for diseases. They are used as the means of modifying the circulation of the blood and, by the auxiliary power thus derived, of securing the more special and desired effects of movements for other regions of the body. When a derivative effect is desired from movements of the region of the feet, it is best secured by employing the auxiliary influence of movements of this region. It must be remembered that every part of the body is charged with the duty of perfecting the circulation of the blood and aiding its passage with in the blood vessels both to and from other parts.

WALKING—This most common and most useful type of exercise is performed chiefly, though not entirely, by the muscles of the legs. The act of walking constitutes a movement that deserves attention, in that it is not only an element in many of these prescriptions, but also is frequently prescribed by physicians.

The exercise of walking is extremely gentle and it becomes fatiguing only by being unduly prolonged. The leg is raised, not by direct lifting, but by causing of the limb to deviate from the vertical by simply bending the thigh and knee joints. This action shortens the distance between the hip and foot, and thus the foot is elevated from the ground. requiring comparatively little muscular power. Then the leg is brought forward, not by projecting it by means of sheer muscular force, but by an easy swinging motion, like that of a pendulum, its own momentum assisting the action. The progress of the trunk, in the forward direction renders the swinging of the leg necessary and easy.

In walking, all muscles of the legs and feet are moderately exercised, as are those of the back and shoulders. Through the action of the latter the body is kept upright, while the arms gently swing with a motion opposite to that of the legs, so as to preserve the center of gravity over the changing base. If the pace is quickened, the muscles of the feet and legs begin a more vigorous action. This great expenditure of muscular power calls for more rapid and deeper respiration and the respiratory muscles respond energetically to the demand; the chest dilates and air passes into the farthest cells of the lungs.

In consequence of these actions, an excess amount of heat is developed. More water, carbonic acid, and urea are produced, and these soon show up at the different bodily outlets; perspiration appears upon the surface of the whole skin, there are more frequent calls for urination, and the volume of vapor discharged by the lungs is greatly increased.

Walking is doubtless superior to any other single exercise that a person can take, yet it fails to answer all the ends of exercise. As there are many other exercises better adapted to preserve the health and power of all the organs of the well man, so there are others better adapted to certain diseased conditions. Walking alone fails to bring the abdominal organs into sufficient activity. On the contrary, these organs are simply carried and are—until the respiration becomes accelerated—nearly as inactive as when the body is resting. Hence weakened persons complain of a dragging sensation while walking and without some other movement to invigorate the diseased parts, walking may be considered not only useless, but even injurious to the health. In these cases, certain movements of the trunk and abdomen are absolutely necessary to render walking proper and useful.

9. Wing-Stride-Standing

POSITION—The hands are placed upon the hips, while standing with the back against a smooth wall, the heels two or two-and-a-half feet apart, and five or six inches from the wall, the toes turned outward.

ACTION—First the feet stretch up onto the toes, then the knees bend forward and outward, while the trunk sinks down to the crouch position. Then knees straighten, raising the body to its utmost height. Finally the heels sink and rest upon the floor. At each stage the movement should be performed very slowly, observing a few moments pause between its distinct positions. The movement may be repeated four or five times.

EFFECT—The action is felt at the bottoms of the feet, in the calves of the legs, and, after the knees bend, strongly in all the muscles of the legs. The effect increases in proportion as the knees deviate from the perpendicular by the bending of the knee joints. In the extreme position, the muscles of the perineum, and even of the rectum, are strongly affected.

10. Knee Bending

POSITION—One hand is placed upon the hips, the other rests on some object to steady the body. The trunk is erect, with one leg straight, the foot resting on the floor, and the other leg bent at the knee at a right angle.

ACTION—First the heel on the floor is raised so that the body's weight rests upon the toes. The knee of the same leg slowly bends, and the trunk sinks as low as the leg is able to support it. Then it is again straightened until the trunk returns to its erect position, as the heel sinks back down to the floor. This action should be repeated three or four times with each leg.

EFFECT—This is similiar to that of the leg-swinging movement in the previous chapter. However, in this case the whole weight of the body is supported by one leg and the movement is thereby made much more positive.

11. Balance-Standing

POSITION—One hand is placed in contact with some firm object to steady the body; the other is placed upon the side. With the trunk erect and its weight borne by one foot resting upon a stool about eighteen inches high, the other foot is left to hang free.

ACTION—First the knee slowly bends, lowering the trunk, although the hanging foot does not touch the floor. Then the bent knee is slowly straightened until the body is in the first position. Repeat the action five or six times with each side.

EFFECT—This movement is simply a modification of the previous one, and the effect is much the same.

12. Kneeling, Knee-Stretching

POSITION—While kneeling on a cushion, the hands are placed upon the hips. The heels are prevented from rising by some firm object such as the frame of a sofa.

ACTION—First the trunk inclines forward gently and slowly without bending at the hips or in the back, and with the knees only slightly straightened or stretched. Next the trunk rises upward and backward until it regains its erect position. This movement should be repeated five or six times.

EFFECT—This movement powerfully affects the muscles and connective tissue of the thigh, its influence extending to the hips and back, and to the calves of the legs. It is derivative, and counteracts the ill effects of too much exercise of the front thigh muscles.

13. Leg-Twisting

POSITION—The hands are placed on the hips, the weight rests upon one foot, the other foot is placed upon a slight elevation, diagonally front and about two feet distant.

ACTION—By a slight effort of the body and of the leg upon which it rests, the trunk turns in a horizontal plane upon the axis of the leg, alternately right and left. Care should be taken not to twist so strongly, as to tax the knee joint. The twisting should be performed five or six times each way on each leg.

EFFECT—The amount of contraction of the muscles of the leg in this movement is comparatively small. However, all the muscles together with all the other structures of the part are strongly affected by it. The muscles, nerves, areolar structures, vessels, etc., are subjected to an unusual agitation that induces peculiar sensations and marked effects.

14. Wing Walk, Forward-Fall-Standing

POSITION—The hands are placed on the hips and one foot is placed about two-and-a-half feet ahead of the other in a walking position, the rear foot is at right angles to it.

ACTION—First the heel of the forward foot rises at the same time that the knee slowly bends. Since this action shortens the forward leg, the body is inclined, throwing its weight forward upon it. The bent knee then slowly extends, and the leg becomes straight until the heel reaches the floor, and the trunk is returned to its original position. The action may be repeated five or six times with each leg.

EFFECT—This movement very strongly affects all the muscles of the legs, and it proves derivative in cases of cold feet or rush of blood to the head.

15. Leg-Clapping (Passive)

POSITION—The one foot is placed on a chair or stool, while the weight rests on the other leg with the trunk in an erect or gently reclining posture.

ACTION—With the palms open and fingers outstretched, both hands clap the leg from hip to ankle. The clapping consists of rapid but light strokes of the palms of the hands. Each leg may be clapped throughout its length five or six times. The clapping is a passive movement for the legs, although the arms are active in applying it.

EFFECT—This action imparts a high degree of nervous sensibility to the legs, and greatly increases the vascularity and warmth of the skin. It is derivative not only for the superior organs, but also for the interior vessels. This movement is also an excellent means of warming cold hands and increasing the circulation in the arms.

Region of the Hips

This region includes the pelvis, its contents, and its connections. In debilitation of any cause, this region frequently presents some severe symptoms and is often afflicted with such disease as constipation, prolapse of the womb and rectum, uterine congestion, ovaritis, amenorrhea, leucorrhea, and diseases of the prostate, bladder and sexual organs.

The movements applicable to this region are numerous and important, and give us a means of controlling the circulation and nutrition of these parts, and if well-selected and applied in proper connection with others that may be indicated, they prove an invaluable means for maintaining health.

Most of the following movements necessarily affect the thigh, back, and abdomen because the muscles involved are attached to an extremity in one or the other of these regions. Many of them affect the legs along with the pelvis.

16. Leg Stretching

POSITION—The hands are on the hips, and the body is erect, in a sitting position on the edge of a chair or stool, with the thighs separated at right angles, feet on the floor.

ACTION—First one foot is raised a few inches from the floor. The knee is slowly stretched until the leg is quite straight and, horizontal, pointing diagonally forward. Then the knee bends and the leg returns to its original position. This movement may be repeated five or six times with each limb.

EFFECT—This movement requires strong action of the internal muscles of the pelvis, and of the muscles of the abdomen and upper portion of the leg, and causes the blood to circulate toward the feet. It strengthens the pelvis and is derivative in decongestion of its organs.

17. Knee Stretching

POSITION—With one hand extended and grasping some firm object and the other on the hip, the body stands erect on one foot; the other leg is bent at both knee and hip with the thigh horizontal.

ACTION—First the bent knee is slowly stretched until the leg is straight. Then the knee bends and the leg resumes the original position. This action may be repeated three or four times with each side.

EFFECT—The action in this movement is like that of the preceding, though somewhat more energetic and more difficult to perform, and it produces similiar effects.

18. Knee Raising

POSITION—The hands are placed on the hips, the trunk reclining on a chair or couch with the shoulders a good deal elevated. The feet are on the floor, and the knees are bent at right angles.

ACTION—First the knees are slowly raised, still bent, as high as possible, the lower part of the leg remaining in the same relative position. Then the legs are slowly returned to the original position. This action may be repeated five or six times.

EFFECT—In this action the lower abdominal muscles

and the internal pelvic muscles are strongly affected. The movement strengthens the part and removes internal congestion of the pelvic organs.

19. Leg Forward-Raising

POSITION—The body is steadied with one hand while the other is placed on the hip. The body is in a standing position, with the weight on one leg.

ACTION—The non-supporting leg is raised slowly forward to the horizontal; then it is slowly returned to its original position. This action may be repeated four or five times with each leg.

EFFECT—This is similiar to that of the preceding movement.

20. Leg Backward-Raising

POSITION—This is the same as in the previous movement.

ACTION—The free leg is extended slowly backward and raised as high as possible then slowly returned to its first position.

EFFECT—In this movement the muscles of the buttocks, the lower portion of the back, and of the pelvis are strongly affected. It is useful in strengthening these parts and removing internal weakness and congestion. The action of the muscles in the direction in which the leg moves is concentric, while that of the anterior and internal muscles is eccentric.

21. Leg Sideways-Raising

POSITION—This is the same position as in the previous movement.

ACTION—The free leg is slowly raised sideways as far as possible then lowered slowly to its original position.

EFFECT—It is similiar to that of the preceding movement, except that the muscles of the thigh and hip on the side moved are brought into strong action.

Each of the above four movements acts upon the muscles of the thigh and leg in a very powerful manner, especially if the position is maintained for a few moments. Since not only the muscles of the hips and thighs, but also those of the leg, enter into these actions, they are all strongly derivative in their effects.

22. Head-Support, Leg-Raising

POSITION—The head rests upon the folded arms placed upon some object of convenient height—a table or mantlepiece. The feet are on the floor, far back from the support, and the body is held as straight as possible to form a forty-five degree angle with the floor.

ACTION—One leg is slowly raised as high as possible, held for a few moments, then it slowly returned to its first position. The dotted outline of figure 5 indicates the direction and extent of the movement. This action may be repeated four or five times with each leg.

EFFECT—The muscles of the thigh, leg, buttocks,

perineum, and back are strongly affected, as are those of the anterior surface of the body. This movement is especially valuable for sedentary people whose legs have become weak from lack of exercise.

23. Half-Standing, Leg Rotation

POSITION—One hand steadies the body, the other is on the hip. The body is erect, and resting on the leg nearest the supporting hand.

ACTION—The free leg is rotated so that the foot describes the broadest possible circle without hitting the supporting foot. See figure 6. This motion is produced by the alternate gentle action of the muscles attached to the hips. The rotation may be performed six or eight times with each leg.

EFFECT—This movement gently affects all the muscles of the thigh and the centrifugal effect that results from the circular motion restrains the return of the venous circulation for a moment. Consequently, the circulation of the leg is quickened and the leg warmed.

24. Double Leg-Twisting

POSITION—The hands are on the hips, and the trunk is seated upright on a chair. The legs are extended across another chair so that the feet project freely and are placed far enough apart that the toes will barely touch in the movement.

ACTION—First the legs slowly rotate, the toes turning outward, the rotation being effected at the upper extremity of the thigh. They then rotate inward, till the toes touch in a nearly horizontal position. This action is repeated five or six times, in both directions. Care should be taken that the limbs turn on their own axis—without bending at the knees, stretching at the ankles, or in any other way deviating from the original position of the legs.

EFFECT—This movement is chiefly effected by the small muscles around the top of the thigh bone, some of which are closely related to the cavity of the pelvis. It circulates the blood in the legs, strengthens the hips, and removes congestion of the pelvic organs.

25. Lying, Knee-Stretching

POSITION—The hands are placed on the hips and the trunk is resting on its back. The legs are half-bent at both the thigh and knee joints and the feet rest on the same horizontal plane as the back.

ACTION—The knees are slowly straightened, the feet raised and the lower legs aligned with the thigh. The thigh is held at an angle of about forty-five degrees to the body. The position is maintained for a few moments. Then the knees slowly bend, bringing the feet back to their orginal position on the couch. This action may be repeated six or eight times.

EFFECT—If the extreme position of the legs is maintained, the action at the lower portion of the abdomen and in the pelvis is powerful. The anterior part of the leg is also affected.

26. Trunk-Lying, Leg Raising

POSITION—The hands are placed on the crown of the head and the trunk is reclined on a couch. The legs, from the hips down, are projecting beyond the edge of the couch. Their weight will keep them lower than the couch.

ACTION—The legs are slowly raised until they are in a position approaching right angles with the trunk, and are held there for a few moments. Then they are lowered slowly back to their original position. This action may be repeated five or six times.

EFFECT—This movement acts upon the abdominal coverings and the muscles of the pelvis. It presses the pelvic and abdominal contents upward and eccentrically affects the muscles of the chin and hips.

27. Legs-Separation

POSITION—The trunk is resting on its back and the hands are placed on the hips, the head slightly elevated. The legs are raised to approximately the position shown by the dotted line in figure 7.

ACTION—The legs are slowly separated as widely as possible, being carried apart laterally by their own weight. Then they are slowly brought together again. This may be repeated five or six times.

EFFECT—The insides of the legs, the perineum, the pelvis, and the lower portion of the abdomen are affected by this movement.

28. Sidewise-Lying Leg-Raising

POSITION—The body is stretched out on one side horizontally. The head is pillowed on the under arm, while the other hand is placed on the hip.

ACTION—The upper leg is slowly raised as far as possible, held for a few moments, then slowly returned to its original position. This action may be repeated six or eight times on each side.

EFFECT—The sides, the outsides of the legs and hips, and the perineum are brought into action in this movement.

29. Lying, Legs-Rotation

POSITION—This is the same as in movement 26.

ACTION—Holding the legs together and moving form the hips, the feet describe as wide a circle as possible. Then the direction of the rotation is reversed. This change is repeated three or four times.

EFFECT—This movement acts on all the muscles of the thighs and hips, the lower portion of the abdomen and back, also the rectum, uterus, bladder and lower portion of the spinal cord.

30. Reclining, Knee-Stretching

POSITION—The arms are in wing position with the trunk reclining and the shoulders elevated. The legs are bent at right angles at both the thigh and knee joints, the feet resting on the same horizontal level as the body.

ACTION—The knees slowly straighten, without changing the position of the thighs, lifting the feet until the legs are straight. Then the knees slowly bend and the feet return to their original position. This action may be repeated five or six times. The dotted outline in figure 7 shows the position at the end of the first part of the movement.

EFFECT—This movement brings into action all the anterior muscles of the leg, as well as those of the lower abdominal and pelvic regions, and affects the internal organs of these parts. It also warms the feet.

31. Thigh-Rotation

POSITION—The hands are placed on the hips, the trunk reclines backward, and the shoulders and head are elevated. The thighs are bent strongly upon the abdomen, with the knees also bent to their sharpest angle.

ACTION—The knees are revolved five or six times in as broad a circle as possible perpendicular to the body. The direction of the rotation should change four or five times.

EFFECT—This movement enlivens the rectum, lower intestines, and abdominal contents generally. It also strengthens the muscles around the hips, and all the organs depending for their innervation at the lower part of the spinal cord.

32. Spine Knocking

POSITION—In a standing position, one hand is used to steady the body and the trunk leans forward.

ACTION—The free arm and hand, strongly clenched, are used to deal twenty or thirty smart blows upon the lower portion of the spine.

EFFECT—This movement makes a vibratory impression upon the sacral bone and its nerves—the lower portion of the spinal cord and branches. The effect is also communicated to all the pelvic organs—rectum, uterus, bladder, etc.—as a result of the excitement produced in the part of the spinal cord supplying the affected region with nerves.

15 Single Movements: The Trunk.

The trunk of the body is filled with the organs of digestion and respiration, and their appendages. This space is divided into two parts or chambers by the diaphragm: the chamber below the diaphragm containing the apparatus for the digestion of food and the preparation of nutritive material, that above it being devoted to the aeration and circulation of the blood.

There is an intimate connection between these two sets of functions, both physiologically and pathologically. The therapeutic indications also relate to both sets of organs and their functions—even though the symptoms of which the invalid chiefly complains may relate more to one or the other.

There can be no good digestion with imperfect respiration, and no efficient respiration while the blood is overwhelmed with the crude materials derived from imperfect digestion.

Through the process of digestion, solid food is reduced to a fluid state; it then passes from the digestive boundaries into the blood. The circulatory system carries these materials to the lungs, where they become aerated with

the oxygen of respiration, and the products of this reaction are then applied to all the blood plasma being
circulated to the tissues as needed by various vital bodily
requirements.

It has already been shown that the body's health depends upon the manner in which these preparatory processes are performed. The ways of attempting to control
these processes are as numerous as the devices of medicine.

Movements For Aiding The Digestive Organs—It has
already been shown how necessary movements are to
further the different stages of the digestive processes,
set the blood in healthful motion and rouse to activity
the secretory functions, etc.

1. In the alimentary canal we have a tube more than
twenty-five feet in length—variously convoluted and
folded upon itself—the greatest portion of which is quite
free to move when acted upon by external causes. It is
fixed to the abdominal wall by only a few movable attachments, so that it readily yields to the least mechanical
force exerted upon it. The tendency of the several portions of the canal to glide upon each other is facilitated
by their exceedingly smooth and polished surface, lu-
bricated with mucous secretions. These surfaces glide
and play upon each other with every change of posture,
and with the muscular exertion in nearly every part of
the body. These mechanical movements, caused by external sources, give the intestines the stimulus necessary
to induce their characteristic wormlike motion, which
is effected by means of the circular muscle fibers of the
tube itself. It is through this motion that the contents

of the canal are carried forward, enabling the absorption of nutrient fluids and the passage of blood in the direction of the liver.

It is a curious and interesting fact that children and young animals—whose desires for motion are inherent—are inclined to those kinds of exercise and position that necessarily stimulate the abdominal contents described above. It is with exercises such as climbing, rolling, crawling, jumping, and playing that the contents are activated; but we never hear that these movements, though often violent, result in harmful consequences. On the contrary, these are the means that nature prescribes to secure healthful development and power in these essential parts of the body.

2. To insure these healthful effects, nature has provided respiration as an efficient and constant means by which to secure these motions of the alimentary canal. The abdominal contents may be considered as located between two great muscular organs—the diaphragm and the abdominal walls. These muscles act simultaneously upon all the included parts, causing them to play incessantly upon each other and subjecting them to a constant and gentle pressure.

Any deterioration in the body's health diminishes the amount of this motion for the simple reason that in chronic diseases of every kind the respiration is less vigorous than in health. In disease these natural movements are not only less in extent, but faulty in kind, and respiratory movements to the abdominal contents are partially lost. The common causes producing these injurious results are standing or sitting for too long in fixed positions. A style of dress that limits the movements of the chest and abdomen and compresses and weakens the muscles can also produce disastrous consequences.

3. One prime effect of exercise is the increase of the substance and contractability of the abdominal muscular coverings. In the absence of proper exercise, the walls of the abdomen become weak, flabby, and unnaturally distended. When this occurs, the abdominal contents necessarily obey the laws of gravity, become dislocated, and their function consequently impeded. Well-directed movements restore the power of these walls; the sinking organs are reinstated to their original positions and their functions recovered.

4. The action of these muscles necessarily calls blood into them to supply their nutrient needs. The advantage of this does not stop with the maintaining of the powers of these muscles. An equal benefit is derived in the scattering of the visceral congestion, which will necessarily occur when the blood is not used in external parts. Congestion of the mucous surfaces, or of some portion of the glandular apparatus, is quite sure to accompany these weaknesses.

Diseased conditions occur in nearly all forms of dyspepsia, constipation, bronchial, laryngeal and liver afflictions when there is insufficient respiration and inadequate movements of the digestive organs. Often, it is the symptoms which are treated instead of the underlying diseases themselves. In order to correct all of the above-mentioned difficulties, it is only necessary to employ movements with due reference to the pathology of the case, and with a rational understanding of the limits of their

ability to correct physiological aberrations. Otherwise
employed, movements are as likely to do injury as good.
In congestion of the liver, for instance, it is highly improper to employ movements that tend to promote
congestion in a healthy person. Ignorance will not shield
one from the consequences resulting from foolish practice. The beginner cannot be too cautious in prescribing
movement therapy for himself.

Movements For Aiding the Respiratory Organs—The
function of aerating the blood might seem to be more
important than any other of the system. When respiration becomes defective or inefficient—whether from external or internal causes—all other functions speedily
fail. This fact emphasizes the direct dependence of all
other functions upon respiration. All actions in the system, whether sensorial, intellectual, or muscular, require oxygen in the blood, as obtained from the air
through respiration. It is oxygen that reduces the complex compounds into simpler, less noxious forms which
are readily eliminated from the body. It is the abundant
supply of this element—secured by wholesome labor or
by special exercises—that gives the system its healthy
elasticity and tone; withdraw this element by reducing
respiratory capacity, and important vital changes are interrupted, and the forces of the system begin to fail.

The system needs a great amount of oxygen; without
it all parts are equally liable to suffer. Hence all organs
and tissues, including the nerves and muscles, unite in
a common effort to secure it, and to perfect the respiratory process. This is proven by many symptoms in
acute disease. In these cases the efficiency of the res-

piratory process is first diminished by a deterioration of the quality of the blood, whose attraction for oxygen is thereby lessened. The whole system is then aroused, and the respiratory and circulatory actions excited in an effort to attain more air to reduce the noxious carbonic acid, urea and water products to a more neutral state. There are two principal circumstances that control the amount of oxygen received into the system. One is the affinity of the blood and tissues for this element, which varies with the individual's health, habits, diet, etc. The other is the capacity of the chest in terms of volume, and the degree of the mobility of its walls. In good health there is complete harmony between the chemical and mechanical needs of the system for oxygen. But it is also necessary that in health there should be a large surplus capacity, beyond the ordinary needs of supply, to meet the unexpected demands of emergencies which the system may face; for instance, the extra breathing made necessary during temporary forced labor or excessive cold. The powers of the system succumb under such hardships if this reserve capacity for respiration is limited or deficient, as it is in pulmonary afflictions.

It is apparent from anatomical considerations that the walls of the chest are very mobile and well adapted to contain different quantities of air according to circumstances. This cavity is bounded below by a thin muscle—the diaphragm—which is convex upward during respiration, but which when contracted is flattened, leaving much space above it to be filled with air, which simultaneously rushes in to fill the vacuum thus produced.

The sides of the chest are formed by ribs and their tendonous and muscular attachments. The ribs extend downward and forward from the spinal columns and are connected to the sternum in front by long elastic cartilages, except the two lower ribs of each side, whose anterior extremities are entirely free. With the contraction of the diaphragm, the external respiratory muscles simultaneously contract. This action elevates the forward extremities of the ribs, causing them to include a larger space; it also turns them slightly outward, thus contributing to the same result. The extent of this effect is precisely in direct proportion to the degree of the muscular action. It may be inferred that not only is the amount of air contained in the lungs dependent upon the amount of motion of the walls of the chest, but also that the amount of air in the lungs depends upon the tone of these muscular walls.

Habitual immobility of the walls of the chest is a characteristic of all chronic diseases; the capacity of the chest becomes restricted and the power of the muscles lessened. In these cases, the occupations and habits of the individual's lifestyle have not enforced the exercise requirements demanded by the system. In most cases, the evil is not lack of exercise, but the lack of suitable exercises designed to serve the wants of a particular function. The kinds of exercise that weakened and sedentary individuals are most inclined to engage in do not sufficiently affect the respiratory apparatus.

All exercise of the voluntary muscles causes an increase in respiration. Preliminary to any strong muscular efforts an involuntary preparation is made by a deep inspiration.

At such times, the inspired air is frequently held and subjected to all the pressure that the chest can exert upon it, apparently to accelerate and increase the solution of the oxygen brought into contact with the blood. Thus we see that exercise not only increases the expansibility of the chest, but provides blood with a larger supply of oxygen.

Great caution is indispensible in prescribing movements designed to enlarge the chest, for injury can easily result. Weakened persons need to be especially careful of indiscriminate movements. Movements of this region tend to produce congestion. However, movements can also be prescribed to overcome it if it already exists.

The same act that causes the chest to become filled with air, assists the flow of venous blood to the same locality. Hence, movements should always be given to counteract this effect. Failing to do this may increase congestion and even threaten serious hemorrhages.

33. Short-Sitting, Forward-Falling

POSITION—The arms are raised close to the ears and parallel to each other. The trunk is erect, supported upon the edge of seat with the thighs apart at right angles and the feet on the floor so as to form a wide base.

ACTION—The trunk is lowered slowly, diagonally forward over one thigh, bringing the breast in close contact with the knee. It is then slowly raised to the first position. This action may be repeated five or six times on each side.

If it seems advisable that less effort be expended in this movement, the arms may be put in wing position instead of stretch. When considerable effort is demanded, the stretch may be used with weights, such as a pair of dumb-bells in the hands.

EFFECT—This movement affects the region of the loins and, if weights are used, also the back and arms.

34. Short-Sitting, Backward-Falling

POSITION—This is like that in the previous movement, except that it may be necessary to hold the feet down under some firm object.

ACTION—The trunk is to be twisted toward the knee on one side. It is then lowered slowly backward until it is nearly horizontal, where it is held for a few moments. Then the trunk is slowly raised again to the original position. This action may be repeated three or four times with each side.

EFFECT—This movement powerfully calls into action the muscles of the abdomen upon either side, and strengthens them as well as the fasciae of the groin and legs, especially in those regions liable to rupture. It also presses the bowels, and is derivative in respect to the visceral organs.

35. Stretch-Sitting, Backward-Falling

POSITION—This is the same as in the previous movement including the support necessary for the feet.

ACTION—The trunk is lowered directly and slowly back until it is nearly horizontal. It is then raised slowly until it regains the original position. This action may be repeated four or five times.

EFFECT—This is a very useful movement to increase the nutrition of the abdominal coverings, especially the lower portion of the walls of the abdomen. It also produces strong derivative effects, and consequently tends to relieve visceral congestion, and restore the contained organs to their natural locations in the abdominal cavity. If the arms are in wing position, the movement will be easier; if weights are held, it will be even more positive in its effect.

36. Sitting, Trunk Sidewise-Bending

POSITION—One hand is placed on the hips while the arm of the other is stretched straight up. The trunk sits erect, with the thighs apart at right angles, feet extended and braced against the floor.

ACTION—The trunk gently bends at the lumbar region in the direction of the hip upon which the hand is fixed, while the stretched arm retains its position relative to the head. The trunk is lowered as far as possible without raising the buttocks at the opposite side, then slowly returned to its original position. This action may be repeated three or four times upon each side. The extent of the movement will increase after a little practice. If the action needs to be stronger, a weight may be held in the upright hand. The action may be repeated four or five times with each side.

EFFECT—This movement strongly affects the sides of the body, and the effect is extended to the liver, spleen, and other visceral organs.

37. Sitting, Trunk Twisting

POSITION—This is the same as in the previous movement.

ACTION—The trunk remains perpendicular and twists on its own axis while the buttocks remains immovable on the chair or stool. In twisting, the side of the raised arm moves forward, while the opposite side moves to an equal extent backward, about a quarter of a circle, and remains there for a few moments. The trunk then untwists, and returns to the original position. This action may be repeated four or five times with each side.

EFFECT—In twisting movements the limits of the motion are soon reached due to the confined condition of the muscles. Yet this class of movements is potent, especially in the effect on the circulation, nearly all the muscles of the part are put into action—some concentrically, others eccentrically. The muscles produce pressure upon the blood vessels and nerves, followed by an increased flow of blood into, and nutrition of, the parts subjected to this action. Twisting also tends to contract the diameter of the cavity of the trunk, and hence produces slight pressure upon the contained organs. This class of movements is derivative.

38. Change-Twisting

POSITION—The hands are locked upon the top of the head and in all other respects the position is identical with that in the last four examples.

ACTION—The trunk turns on its axis with moderate rapidity as far as possible in alternating directions. This action may be repeated fifteen or twenty times successively.

EFFECT—This movement, for the great majority of the parts affected, is nearly passive; only a few muscles are being employed to give the motion, and all the organs contained in the cavity of the body are agreeably stimulated by the agitation. The movement is tranquilizing for the nerves and equalizing in its effect on the circulation, while certain muscles in different portions of the body are also activated.

39. Sitting, Trunk-Swaying

POSITION—The arms are extended horizontally, trunk sitting, legs apart, and feet well braced.

ACTION—The trunk turns on its own axis but, due to the position of the arms, the action is more deliberate. It turns as far as it can, first in one direction, then the other.Considerable momentum is acquired and this increases the effect of the movement on the loins. This twisting may be repeated ten or fifteen times each way.

EFFECT—The muscles of the top of the shoulders and nearly all those of the arms and sides are strongly affected. The centrifugal effect upon the circulation of the blood in the arms is to detain and then quicken the circulation, and warm the hands. The movement acts derivatively for the chest.

40. Kneeling, Trunk Backward-Bending

POSITION—The arms are stretched upward, parallel with each other and the head. The trunk is erect, in a kneeling position with the knees placed far apart and resting on a cushion.

ACTION—The trunk bends slowly backward from the waist, as far as possible, where it remains for a few moments. It then slowly returns to its original position. The knees and hips remain fixed.

EFFECT—This movement stretches the skin, fasciae and muscles of the anterior portion of the body and legs. It is felt in the groin, the walls of the abdomen, and chest, elevates the ribs, diaphragm, and the visceral contents, and expands the chest. The action is chiefly produced by the muscles of the back, which it strengthens.

This and many other back-bending movements frequently cause sharp sensations in the back, especially at the beginning of their use. This is not because the muscles of that region are strained unduly by the movement. The sensation is produced by the pinching of the vertebral cartilages caused by the unusual position. The sensation gradually eases as the cartilages become more elastic, and as the parts adapt themselves to the new demands required of them. If movements of this class produce an unpleasant tenderness, they must be discontinued for a short time.

VARIATIONS—1. The arms may be in the shelter position instead of stretch. In this case the action is not so forcible and is, therefore, better adapted to those who are quite feeble.

2. The arms are extended exactly as in the swaying movement, but may grasp a couple of weights, such as a pair of dumbells. The effect then becomes much greater, since the added weight acts powerfully upon the whole anterior surface of the body through the leverage of the arms and body.

3. While the arms are in either of the above positions, the legs may be placed in walking position, that is, with one knee ahead of the body, the other behind it, both as far apart as convenient. In this case, after the action has been repeated three or four times, the position of the legs may be reversed. The action is now felt much more powerfully in the groin, and the movement is especially useful in strengthening the muscles and fasciae around the hernial region.

41. Kneeling Trunk-Twisting

POSITION—One arm is extended upward, while the hand of the other is placed upon the hip. The trunk is erect in the kneeling position with the legs widely apart.

ACTION—The side of the extended arm moves forward while the opposite side moves backward, twisting the body upon its axis. This action is to be repeated four

or five times with each side. It should be remembered
that in this movement the position is that of kneeling,
with the body bent a little backward.

EFFECT—This movement is felt at the sides and in
the arm which is in stretch position, and across the abdomen at the lower abdominal cavity, strengthening
these regions as well as acting derivatively.

42. Walk-Kneeling, Trunk Twisting

POSITION—One arm is stretched upward, the hand
of the other being on the hips. The trunk erect in the
kneeling position. The knee on the same side with the
stretched arm is placed as far back as is possible, the
opposite knee as far forward.

ACTION—The side of the stretched arm moves forward, while the opposite side moves backward, twisting
the body on its axis as far as practicable. After this motion
has been repeated four or five times, the knee positions,
are reversed and the motion is repeated as before.

EFFECT—This movement acts strongly upon the abdominal muscles and fasciae—especially those of the
groin—and increases the power and resistance of those
parts.

43. Kneeling, Arm Stretching

POSITION—The arms are in angle position, with the
elbow bent and the upper part of the arms near the side

of the body. The trunk is kneeling, knees far apart and thighs leaning back from the perpendicular.

ACTION—The arms are slowly stretched upward until they become parallel, where they remain for a short time. They then slowly return to the original position. This may be repeated six or seven times. In figure 8, the dotted line shows the position after the first part of the movement, the extreme position. Care should be taken that the arms are not stretched perpendicularly, but exactly in line with the leaning trunk.

EFFECT—The parts affected by this movement are the arms, the tops of the shoulders, the region beneath the shoulder blades, the sides of the chest, the diaphragm, and the abdominal muscles, as well as the visceral organs, which are raised by it and moderately compressed.

VARIATIONS—1. The hands may grasp some heavy objects, such as a pair of dumbbells, which increases the effect upon all of the parts mentioned.

2. The legs may be in walking position. In this case the effect upon the abdomen, especially upon the groin, is much increased.

44. Arms Backward-Striking

POSITION—The arms are in rack position, leaning slightly back extended horizontally forward. The trunk is in kneeling position and knees apart.

ACTION—The arms are thrown horizontally backward as far as possible. This action is repeated eight or ten times.

EFFECT—There are only a few muscles brought into active play in this movement, and these are situated back of the shoulder. By this movement the muscles of the breast are acted upon, the ribs elevated, and the blood forced into the hands, increasing their warmth. This movement may be practiced slowly; if done quickly, an increased effect is produced upon the anterior muscles.

45. Stride-Kneeling, Sidewise Swaying

POSITION—The hands are placed on the hips. The trunk is perpendicular and kneeling, legs in stride position.

ACTION—The trunk bends to one side from the waist as far as it can. It then returns and passes through the perpendicular for the same distance on the opposite side. The motion is somewhat rapid so that the momentum acquired will be felt upon the convex side. This action may be repeated ten or twelve times. Flexibility and the amount of practice will determine the extent of the motion.

EFFECT—This movement acts upon the muscles of either side, and also upon the liver, spleen, and other organs situated in the region affected by the motion, as well as the abdominal walls and viscera.

VARIATIONS—1. The arms may be in stretch position. The motion then is much more slowly performed, and the effect much greater, while at the same time more gentle.

2. The arms may be in stretch position, the hands

grasping a pair of weights. This variation adds greatly to the effort, making the movement a gentle and very effective one.

46. Stride-Kneeling, Trunk-Twisting

POSITION—The arms are extended sideways in· a line, palms of the hands downward. The trunk is erect and kneeling, the legs apart in stride position.

ACTION—The trunk turns on its axis as far as the muscles will allow, from right to left, and then from left to right, and so continues, repeating the action of twisting without bending the body, the arms being maintained in the straight line. This may be repeated eight or ten times.

EFFECT—This movement affects the coverings of the abdomen, and the muscles of the back. It also warms the hands, and is derivative for the chest.

47. Arm-Raising

POSITION—The arms hang in their natural position at the sides, trunk erect, sitting, legs in stride position.

ACTION—The arms slowly rise sideways, the backs of the hands uppermost, until the hands meet perpendularly above the head, where they remain for a short time. Then they return slowly to the original position. This action may repeated six or eight times.

EFFECT—In this movement the muscles of the top

of the shoulder, and all of the muscles of the sides of the chest, are brought into action—the former concentrically, the latter eccentrically. The ribs are raised and the diameter of the chest increased. The diaphragm is also affected.

48. Half-Kneeling, Trunk Backward Bending

POSITION—The arms are in upward stretch position, the trunk erect. One leg is kneeling, while the other is extended forward with the sole of the foot on the floor.

ACTION—The trunk bends slowly backward so as to carry the arms, which must be kept parallel with the head and in a straight line with the trunk, as far backward as possible. It slowly resumes the original position. This action may be repeated three or four times, when the position of the legs should be reversed, and the action repeated.

EFFECT—The lower portion of the abdomen, the groin, and the whole anterior surface of the body are affected by this movement. The parts acted upon are strengthened, and those beneath experience a derivative influence.

49. Weight-Held Bending

POSITION—One hand rests on the hips, the foot of the same side is elevated upon a step or a stair. The other hand holds a weight, the forearm resting on the head. The weight of the body, which is erect, is sustained principally by the leg on the floor.

ACTION—The trunk slowly bends at the waist in the direction of the elevated foot, being assisted by the weight in the upper hand. It then returns slowly to the original position. This action may be repeated four or six times with each side of the body.

EFFECT—This movement allows the muscles of the concave side to remain nearly passive—the bending is mostly produced by the weight—while the muscles of the convex side are felt strongly in the stretch. The movement affects the walls of the body on sides, as well as the contiguous internal organs.

50. Step-Standing, Diagonal-Bending

POSITION—In this movement no weight is held, and the arm is in upward-stretch position. In all other respects, the position is precisely like that in the previous movement.

ACTION—The trunk bends as in the previous movement, but it is brought into the curve of the final position by the action of the muscles of the side. The movement is repeated four or five times on each side.

EFFECT—The effects of the movement differ little from those of the previous movement.

51. Step-Standing, Sidewise-Bending

POSITION—One arm is in wing position. The leg of the same side is extended forward in kick position and maintained in place by a stool. The arm of the opposite side is in stretch position, the trunk angles back and rests with its weight on the rear leg.

ACTION—The trunk slowly bends in the direction opposite the stretched arm. Then it returns to the first position.

EFFECT—This movement affects the groin and iliac region of the stretched side.

VARIATION—Both arms may be extended in stretch position, instead of only one. The twisting will then be performed in the same direction as before, with the movement in every respect like the one just described. In this case the movement affects the trunk and elevates the ribs more than in the first.

52. Step-Standing, Trunk Twisting

POSITION—The position is exactly like that in the previous movement.

ACTION—The trunk twists upon its axis, the stretched side moving forward, the opposite side backward and then returns to the original position. This action is repeated four or five times with each side.

EFFECT—This movement affects nearly all the muscles of the body.

53. Long-Sitting, Trunk Forward Bending

POSITION—The hands are placed upon the head in shelter position, the trunk in sitting position. The legs are extended horizontally. The movement should be done on a cushion.

ACTION—The trunk bends slowly forward as far as possible. It returns slowly to the original position. This action may be repeated five or six times.

EFFECT—This movement elevates the ribs, causes the abdominal muscles to contract, elevates the abdominal contents, and effects eccentrically the muscles of the back and buttocks.

54. Half-Standing, Arms Stretching

POSITION—The arms are bent at the elbows, with the upper part of the arm by the side of the body. The trunk angles back with one leg placed two feet forward in kick position, the foot supported by a stool. The weight of the body rests mainly upon the other leg.

ACTION—The arms slowly rise, straightening the elbows and keeping the extending arms in the direction of the transverse plane of the body, until they become straight and parallel with each other. The head is somewhat thrown back. This position is retained for a few moments. The arms then slowly resume the first position. This action may be repeated three or four times, when the position of the legs should be reversed, and the action repeated. The dotted outlines of the arms in figure 9 show the original position and the stretched arms the limit of the upward motion.

EFFECT—In this movement the entire anterior surface of the body and the tops of the shoulders are strongly acted upon, as well as the parts beneath the shoulder blades and the muscles connected with the ribs. It develops the muscles of these regions, is derivative for the chest, and is valuable as a means of assisting in its expansion.

VARIATIONS—1. The same movement can be done holding a pair of dumbbells. This modification of the movement greatly increases its effects.

2. The movement may begin in the stretch position, instead of the angle. The effect in this case will be essentially the same.

55. Walk-Standing, Trunk Twisting

POSITION—One arm is in stretch, the other in wing position. The legs are in walk position with a long distance between the feet, the leg of the wing side being brought forward, and the trunk bent toward the same side.

ACTION—The trunk slowly twists upon its axis, the stretched arm side moving forward and the opposite backward. It then returns to the primary position. This action may be repeated four or five times with each side.

EFFECT—This movement puts the muscles of the sides into powerful eccentric action. It is beneficial in cases of central congestion, and strengthens the chest and abdomen.

56. Walk-Standing, Trunk Backward Bending

POSITION—The arms are extended horizontally on either side, the trunk erect. One foot is placed before, and the other behind, the center of the body and two-and-a-half feet apart.

ACTION—The trunk bends backward as far as it can, where it remains a moment. It then returns to the original position. This action may be repeated three or four times, and then the legs should exchange places, and the action be repeated again.

EFFECT—This movement expands the chest, warms the hands, and strengthens the back.

57. Doorway-Walking

POSITION—This is taken in a doorway, the arms being extended upward and outward with the palms pressed against the frame. The trunk is erect, the feet behind the middle portion of the threshold.

ACTION—One leg is raised as if to walk, but somewhat higher than normal. At the same time the body is projected forward but is arrested by the hands against the door frame so that the center of the trunk is very much curved forward. The raised leg returns to its place beside the other on the floor and at the same time the trunk straightens, resuming the original position. Next the other leg is raised and the sequence attempted there arrested walking repeated. This action may be repeated with each leg ten or twelve times. Figure 10 shows the movement at the point when the raised leg and the projecting trunk are falling back into the original position.

EFFECT—This movement acts powerfully in expanding the chest and tends to develop all the muscles of the front portion of the body. Once learned, it is easily performed and requires little exertion compared to the amount of effect produced. In this respect it very much resembles a true duplicated movement.

58. Standing Trunk Rotation

POSITION—The hands are locked on the top of the head. The trunk is bent to one side, with the legs in stride and the body in standing position.

ACTION—The trunk is made to rotate, carrying the head around a circle of considerable extent. The axis of motion is just above the hips. This rotary motion may be performed three or four times each way, when the trunk should bend to the opposite side to the same extent, and the motion repeated as many times more.

EFFECT—This movement strengthens the parts of the loins, and expands the chest.

VARIATION—This movement may be taken in the sitting position. In this case—the body being more firmly supported—the diameter of the circle described by the head may be greater than while standing. and this will cause greater action of the sides. This movement affects the liver and spleen.

59. Head-and-Heels Lying

POSITION—The trunk lies in a horizontal position, with the hands clasped on the head, the legs parallel. Only the head and the heels rest on supports, such as two chairs, while the remaining portion of the body is suspended (see figure 11).

ACTION—The body remains in this position for a longer or shorter time, according to the individual's strength.

EFFECT—The muscles of the back are forced into powerful action in this movement. Hence it is derivative in respect to the spinal cord, while it increases the development and power of the muscles of the back.

VARIATION—The supports may be placed closer to each other. The movement thereby becomes less powerful, and the holding may continue longer.

60. Elbows-and-Toes Lying

POSITION—The arms are in rack elbow-bent position; the trunk is horizontal, face downward. Only the elbows and toes rest on a mattress (see figure 12).

ACTION—The trunk is held in this position for a few moments, according to the strength of the subject.

EFFECT—This movement produces a muscular tension and contraction of the whole forward part of the body, the effect of which is especially felt at the lower portion of the abdomen. It presses the abdominal contents toward the diaphragm, and often instantly relieves prolapsus on any of the pelvic organs—such as that of the womb, vagina, or rectum—restoring the parts to their natural condition and position. By repetition the weak parts are strengthened, and a radical cure is effected.

VARIATION—While in the position described above, the hips may rise slowly upward, and after a moment, slowly fall to the level of the elbows and toes. This movement may be repeated six or eight times. This way of performing the movement is often more agreeable, as well as somewhat more positive, and produces similiar effects.

61. Sidewise-Lying, Hips Raising

POSITION—One arm lies upon the trunk, while the elbow of the other rests upon a mattress. The trunk is extended horizontally, the lower leg lying with its side upon the mattress, the other resting upon it.

ACTION—The hips are raised slowly upward, and remain lifted for a few moments. Then they return to their first position. This action may be repeated four or five times with each side.

EFFECT—This movement is strongly felt at the side of the hip which is under at the time, and acts throughout the whole side of the body. It also affects the back.

62. Back Lying, Head and Legs Raising

POSITION—The trunk lies horizontally upon the back, supported by a mattress. The hands are clasped upon the head, legs parallel.

ACTION—Both the feet and head are raised from the horizontal at the same time, curving the body, and are held for a short period. Then they return to the original position. This action may be repeated five or six times.

EFFECT—This movement is a very powerful one for the abdominal muscles, derivatively affecting the visceral organs. It also increases the force of the general circulation and urges the blood into the capillaries of the entire system.

VARIATION—Only the back may be supported, instead of the whole length of the body. The effect is similar.

63. Back Lying, Holding

POSITION—The arms remain in contact with the body at the sides. The trunk rests with the back supported by a single chair. The legs, head, and shoulders, unsupported, fall below the horizontal.

ACTION—The body is allowed to remain for a short period in this position.

EFFECT—This is chiefly felt in the front of the body which in this position is stretched, and receives eccentric action. The curved position causes considerable pressure upon the abdominal contents.

64. Trunk Vibration

POSITION—The hands are placed on the hips. The knees and thighs are bent to the greatest possible extent in a crouch, the feet resting on the floor about two feet apart. The trunk is maintained in a position as erect as the position of the legs will allow.

ACTION—The body is slightly raised by the exertion of all the muscles of the legs, on which its weight rests, and is directly permitted to return with the force of its weight to the same position. It should rise only a few inches. Repeat the action a dozen times or more, as fast as possible.

EFFECT—This is felt in the perineum and rectum, exciting its contractability to a noticeable, and sometimes remarkable, degree. This movement encourages the emptying of the bowels in cases of constipation.

65. Abdominal Movements (Passive)

A great variety of motions may be administered to aid one's digestive organs. Each can be adapted to different constitutions, conditions of disease, developments of the region, strengths of the person, etc. A few forms have been selected which, if not applicable for a given case, may prove suggestive of another that may be more appropriate.

POSITION—Lying upon a couch, with the shoulders raised and the legs in an easy position. Alternatively, the position may be standing with the trunk a little stooped.

ACTION—Several variations are possible, as follows:

1. *Kneading*—Two clenched fists may be pressed upon the abdomen firmly so as to cause the underlying organs to react. This action is to be repeated for several

minutes over the whole region of the abdomen. The movement excites the muscular contractability of the intestinal tube and promotes fecal elimination.

2. *Shaking*—The hands are applied to each side of the abdomen, and alternate pressure given to it, producing a somewhat rapid oscillating movement of all the abdominal contents in the area between the hands. This movement promotes venous absorption and removes congestion.

3. *Stroking*—Each hand is applied to the region of the groin, the tips of the fingers nearly meeting. Then each hand is to be drawn slowly across the groin, with pressure extending upward and outward. This movement has an effect similiar to that of kneading.

4. *Circular Stroking*—The pressure of the hands is made to follow the course of the colon, beginning low upon the right side of the abdomen, passing around beneath the stomach, and terminating on the opposite side. This movement also promotes fecal elimination.

5. *Point Pressure*—This may be performed under the short ribs. The ends of the fingers are applied from below, and strong pressure is made with a tremulous motion. The movement excites muscular and nervous action in the adjacent organs and in certain cases relieves pain.

6. *Clapping*—The open hands are made to strike any portion of the frontal regions of the body. The blows should be given with each hand alternately and at such a rate of rapidity and force as to produce no unpleasant sensations. If there is a region where pain is felt, each successive application should, for a period, be given to surrounding parts, approaching the tender part gradually until the pain disappears.

The doubled fist may be used instead of the flat hand. This movement promotes absorption and removes congestion.

EFFECTS—The above motions are adaptations of a few of the duplicated movements that may be applied to the part. Their effects are often highly beneficial.

It is not necessary to do each of these movements in a distinct form, because in every pathological state there is a general similarity of condition to that of other states. The effects above merge with each other as do the applications themselves. With congestion of the mucous membrane, there may be drying and stickiness .Or there may be an attempt at relief by the body through diarrhea. In either case the capillaries need to have their contents forced to flow along their course. In either case, too, the underlying muscles need more nutrition and power. In both, the circulation needs to be equalized, and nutritive absorption produced.

66. Agitation of the Abdomen and Diaphragm

POSITION—Wing-stride-sitting.

ACTION—The abdominal coverings and diaphragm are contracted by strong efforts exerted in rapid succession, producing an oscillatory motion of the entire abdominal contents. This may be continued for several minutes.

EFFECT—This movement promotes the contractile power of all the muscular tissues participating in it, and the functional action of all the organs affected by it.

16 Single Movements: The Arms

The region of the arms is intimately connected with that of the chest. This connection is not only suggested by its contiguity to the chest, but by the anatomical relationship of the parts. The arms are connected to the chest by large and strong muscles spreading themselves over a good portion of its surface. The blood vessels and nerves of the chest also extend along the arms. Thus, the gymnast, who uses his arms vigorously and habitually, never fails to obtain an ample development of the chest.

Several movements have already been described in which very potent effects are incidentally experienced in the arms and hands. Indeed, movements of the chest and arms are so interrelated that no absolute and precise distinction can be drawn between those of the two regions. Power may be exerted by the arms in every direction, and in each of these there will result a distinct effect to both the arms and the chest.

The number of cases in which one arm is stronger than the other are numerous, indicating an unbalanced and partial use of these important members. An arm can become useless from nervous shocks, especially in children, and its growth partly ceases. It can continue to be powerless because the parent or physician does not direct the nutritive actions into the channels in which they are especially needed. These results are conspicious in the arms, but the principle is equally true throughout the body.

In all cases of great weakness, the treatment must be gradual at first and the energies and nutrition of the system must be directed outward. The blood of central congestion needs to be removed to external members deficient in it. The use of arm movements is the proper means of beginning treatment in these cases. In this way the pressure in the large central vessels is relieved, and thereby a most important advantage is gained in the treatment of the disease.

The novice is advised not to neglect this essential portion of the treatment, for diseases situated in the superior cavity of the trunk are the most difficult and dangerous of all under any kind of treatment.

The reader will note that in the examples of movements of the lower extremities, advantage is taken of the weight of the whole body or of some portion of it. The weight is made to act upon the regions to which the movement is principally directed.

67. Stretch Backward-Lying

POSITION—The arms are stretched with the trunk extended upon the back. The crown of the head projects a little beyond the edge of the couch, and weights are held in the hands.

ACTION—The weights are held for a length of time proportionate to the strength of the individual, the action consisting of holding.

EFFECT—The weights not only task the muscles of the undersides of the arms, but the arms serve as levers by whose action the ribs are raised and the chest enlarged. There is little voluntary effort in this movement, but much valuable effect is produced. It is particularly advantageous for strong persons, though useful for the weak, too, if not carried too far.

VARIATIONS—1. The arms may be slowly raised, maintaining their parallel position to each other until they reach the perpendicular, when they are gradually lowered again. This may be repeated six or eight times. This manner of performing the movement is somewhat easier than the first, and produces similiar effects.

2. The arms may describe a horizontal arc on each side, repeating the motion three or four times. This way of employing the movement calls other muscles into play.

68. Rack Grasp, Forward Falling

POSITION—The arms are extended forward, the hands grasping some convenient object, such as a bed or the top of a mantle. The body is in forward-fall-standing position, forming an angle of about forty-five degrees.

ACTION—The elbows slowly bend outward while the body falls forward until the head is brought close to the object of support. The elbows now slowly stretch, bringing the trunk back into the original position. This action may be repeated four or five times. The dotted outline in figure 13 indicates the extent of the movement.

EFFECT—In this movement not only the arms are affected, but the chest is expanded, and the anterior muscles of the abdomen are acted upon.

VARIATION—Some means of support about half as high as that represented in the figure may be employed.

In this case the strain is greater upon the arms and hands, and the influence upon the anterior muscles of the abdomen is increased so as to elevate the ribs and visceral organs.

69. Standing, Hip Rotation

POSITION—The arms are stretched vertically upward to hold a horizontal bar placed eight or ten inches below the point of utmost reach, feet and hands are held close together.

ACTION—The hips bend to one side, and then revolve in a circle, the diameter of which is as extensive as the position of the body will allow. The revolutions are performed eight or ten times in each direction. Figure 14 shows the position, the dots outlining the circle in which the hips revolve.

EFFECT—The hands and arms sustain nearly the whole weight of the body, and the motion affords action alternately to nearly all the muscles of the arms. The same effect is also experienced in nearly equal degrees by the chest, with the ribs being elevated. The size of the chest and the action of the respiratory muscles are increased. The strong tension of the arms also produces a derivative effect upon the chest, and the hands are warmed. There is little exertion of the will expended in this movement and consequently there is little fatigue.

70. Standing, Arm Twisting

POSITION—One arm is stretched upward and the hand grasps a transverse pole placed at a convenient height while the body is standing erect.

ACTION—The trunk turns without moving from its standing-point which, as the grasp of the hand is maintained, causes the arm to be twisted. It then turns in the opposite direction, continuing until the arm is untwisted and twisted again in the opposite direction. This action may be repeated four or five times with each arm.

EFFECT—This movement causes all the muscles of the arm to act strongly and eccentrically. It affects all the blood vessels, small and large, is strongly derivative, and warms the hands.

71. Sitting, Arm Twisting

POSITION—The arms are extended at either side in the same straight line, body in a sitting position.

ACTION—The arms are twisted upon their own longitudinal axis, first forward, then backward, alternately. They may be twisted eight or ten times each way.

EFFECT—This movement engages all the muscles of

the arms in both concentric and eccentric action. It is highly stimulating to the circulation, warms the hands, and is derivative for the chest.

72. Arms Rotating

POSITION—The arms are stretched upward, trunk in the upright standing posture.

ACTION—The arms move from the shoulder joint to describe circles perpendicular to and parallel with the body, the diameters of which are twice the length of the arm. After revolving in one direction ten or a dozen times, the direction is reversed.

EFFECT—This movement causes the blood to be retained in the arms and hands, because the centrifugal force attained by the rotation counteracts the return of venous circulation; at the same time, the arterial flow is assisted. The consequence is that the hands become not only warmed, but absolutely swollen with blood, and the tendency toward cold hands is overcome. The movement also relieves congestion of the chest and affects all the muscles and ligaments around the shoulder joint, including those that are spread across the chest.

VARIATIONS—1. One arm may be in wing position, while the movement is performed by the other arm, with alterations after a suitable number of revolutions. The effect of this way of performing the movement is greater than if both arms revolved at the same time. The body accomodates itself better to the single than to the double movement, and the objective is achieved in a shorter time, and with less tendency to fatigue.

2. The movement may be started in the rack position. One arm may be brought backward as nearly horizontal as possible, with a swinging motion. While it is returning to the original position, the other arm begins the same motion. These alternating motions may be done fifteen or twenty times.

73. Hanging, Swinging

POSITION—For this movement a swing apparatus is necessary: a pole about three feet long, suspended horizontally at each end by ropes and so high that it can just be reached by a person standing upon the floor. The higher the ceiling from which the apparatus is suspended, the greater the arc through which the body swings, and the more desirable the arrangement. The hands grasp the pole.

ACTION—The person springs forward and upward and hangs by the hands. The momentum thus acquired causes pendulum-like swing, the feet describing the arc of a large circle. The motion may be continued as long as the grasp can be sustained.

EFFECT—This motion does not cause fatigue, since the will is only slightly exerted, but the effects are very important. A powerful derivative effect is produced chiefly to the central portions of the body. This comes from the strong actions of the muscles of the hands, arms, and shoulders, required to sustain the body; the prolonged tension produces a rush of the blood into the arms. In addition, the swinging motion, producing a very great centrifugal effect upon the circulating fluids, causes them to flow into the lower extremities and be retained there. In other words, the venous circulation is, for a time, retarded while the arterial is accelerated. The result is an accumulation of blood in the lower extremities, expanding the vessels and increasing the nutrition of that region. While these objectives are being attained, the equally important one of diminishing the amount of blood in central portions of the body is also secured and the circulation is equalized.

Another desirable effect produced by this movement is the elevation of the ribs, with subsequent expansion of the chest. The arms being connected by muscular attachments to the ribs, both before and behind, the body is really suspended at the walls of the chest in such a way as to force them outward, and to allow the inspired air to occupy a larger space.

It is evident that in this movement most of the indi- cations for the treatment of chronic pulmonary afflictions of various types are achieved. The same may be said in respect to the treatment of afflictions of the liver, and the dyspepsia usually associated with it. Hence, for chronic invalids of nearly every class, this is a movement as important as it is easily performed.

74. Trunk Rotation

POSITION—The hands grasp the swing as in the previous movement, but the feet remain on the floor.

ACTION—The body falls to one side by its weight;

being sustained by the swing, it bends at the side or shoulders, while the toes remain on the floor directly under the point of suspension.

ACTION—By a little effort, the body is made to revolve in a circle, the longest diameter of which is at the shoulders, care being taken to keep it constantly facing one way. It may revolve several times in each direction.

EFFECT—In this movement every part of the body's surface is stretched as the weight is thrown upon it and relaxed as the revolution throws the weight upon other muscles. The intercostal muscles of the ribs and those of the arms are particularly subjected to the action, as are the muscles of the abdomen, back, and legs. Since this movement is accomplished with little effort, it is very refreshing. It also develops the chest and respiratory apparatus, and is useful in dissipating the unpleasant feelings of fatigue, or any congestion that may have been produced by the expenditure of too much power in the practice of other movements.

VARIATION—Instead of revolving in a circle, the body may remain stationary at any given point in the circle. For instance, in the furthest forward position the anterior portion of the body is convex—the feet being placed far back—and strong action is produced upon the muscles of the chest and abdomen.

75. Hanging, Holding

POSITION—The hands firmly grasp some object at shoulder height. The feet and legs are extended backward, with the toes resting on the floor. The body takes on a curved shape, the convexity being anterior.

ACTION—The trunk is straightened so that it forms a line diagonal to that of the arms. It's then lowered into its original curved position. This may be repeated two or three times. The dotted outline in figure 15 indicates the starting position, while the solid outline shows the position attained by stretching.

EFFECT—This movement affects the anterior portion of the hands, arms, chest, abdomen, and legs.

VARIATION—The body may take the position shown in the picture and be held there for a few moments. The effects are very similiar to those of the above movement, but perhaps a little more marked. The top of a bedpost or a mantle will provide an adequate support for this movement.

76. Elbows-Support Lying

POSITION—The arms are extended on either side in the yard position and are supported by a chair or cushioned stool under each elbow. The back of the heels are supported by the floor, the body being carefully maintained in the straight line.

ACTION—The position may be maintained for about one minute. Figure 16 shows the position and action.

EFFECT—This movement affects the back of the arms, the muscles between the shoulders and under the shoulder blades, and those of the back. It strengthens all these parts and is derivative for the spinal cord.

77. Half-Standing-Stretching

POSITION—One arm is extended horizontally and, being in contact with some object such as a wall, helps to maintain the upright position of the body. The other arm is stretched upward while the foot of the same side is standing upon a stool. The other leg is free; the trunk is erect.

ACTION—The action in this movement does not consist in change of place, nor in holding, but in tensing all the muscles of the standing side of the body, the action of each muscle being exactly balanced by that of its antagonist. In other words, all of the muscles of one side of the body are stretched by a strong exertion of the will. After the action has continued for a minute on one side, reverse the action to the other side. Figure 17 indicates the position.

EFFECT—This movement is quite fatiguing, and is strongly derivative in its effects. It may be used on one side when that side is much weaker than the opposite, as in hemiplegia, curvature of spine, etc.

78. Standing-Stretching

POSITION—The arms are stretched upward and outward. The legs are in the stride position, trunk erect.

ACTION—An effort is simultaneously made by nearly all the muscles of the body to reach higher, and this action is continued for a full minute.

EFFECT—This is a very fatiguing movement, since

it calls for a powerful exertion of the will to maintain the simultaneous action of so many muscles. The effect is derivative, and equalizing to the circulation and the nervous and nutritive forces.

17 Single Movements: The Head and Neck.

The motions of the head are caused by the action of the muscles of the neck, some of which are attached at the base of the skull and the framework of the chest. The neck contains numerous and powerful muscles, enabling the head to assume an extensive range of positions and to perform a variety of important movements. These movements are useful from a hygenic as well as medical point of view, chiefly because they affect the circulation of the blood to and from the head, and also enable us because they modify, to some extent, the circulation and nutrition of the throat, and several of the sense organs: the eyes, ears, nose, etc. These muscles of the neck are prone to disease or weakness and they are often called upon to assist in removing certain natural and acquired faults of position, or deformities, not only of the neck, but also of the spine.

In treating this region, it is more convenient to refer to the head, since changes in the position of the head accomplish the most noticeable results, even though the neck is the region to which the action is actually applied.

79. Head Turning

POSITION—The body may be in a sitting or standing position with the head erect—the beginning position for all head movements.

ACTION—The head turns upon its axis to the right, as far as possible, and then—in the same manner and to the same extent—to the left. The action may be repeated six or eight times each day.

EFFECT—This movement brings all the muscles of the neck into strong action, so that they press on the blood vessels and aid the circulation in this region.

80. Head Forward Bending

POSITION—This is the same as in the previous movement.

ACTION—The head is bent directly forward as far as it can go, bringing the chin close to the breast. It is then returned to the original position. This action may be repeated six or eight times.

EFFECT—This movement is concentric for the front part of the neck, and eccentric for the back. It is sometimes advantageous, due to its influence on the vertebral vessels, in removing headaches. It is also useful in afflictions of the throat.

81. Head Backward Bending

POSITION—This is the same as in the previous movement.

ACTION—The head is carried backward as far as possible. It then returns to its first position. This action to be repeated six or eight times.

EFFECT—This is nearly the same as that in the head turning. The kind of action, however, is different; the eccentric action is exercised by the anterior muscles, while the concentric is effected by the muscles at the back of the neck.

82. Head Bending and Twisting

POSITION—The same as in the previous movement.

ACTION—The head bends backward. It then turns to the right and then to the left, retaining the back bend and alternating the motion.

EFFECT—This movement acts quite powerfully upon the front of the neck. Its derivative effects are upon the laryngeal mucous membrane in cases of congestion of that surface.

83. Head Twisting

POSITION—The head is bent forward and sidewise.

ACTION—The head slowly bends backward, turning the face upward, while at the same time the head turns upon its axis until it looks toward one shoulder. The motion is like the turning of a screw. The head may be returned to the primary position, and then rise and turn in the opposite direction. This action may be repeated each way five or six times.

EFFECT—This movement is therapeutic in much the same way as those previously described. It is also useful in lateral curvature of the spine, but in this case the turning should be in only one direction.

18   Disease & Holistic Healing

No attempt will be made to delve into the symptoms and progressive stages of the diseases amenable to holistic healing, such an account would swell the size of this volume and defeat its objective. There are many excellent treatises already available about these subjects.

The following chapters will presume knowledge on the part of the reader in regard to the nature and symptoms of the diseases written about. It must be further explained that the exercises contained in this book aim at the correction of the primary causes of disease and regard secondary symptoms as merely effects, consequently demanding less treatment.

The following pages expose the essential nature of certain illnesses in connection with their causes, not in the light of ordinary, orthodox treatment.

The curative process is regarded as physiological in nature, as opposed to the critical and artificial actions that are common to medical practice. These processes have both chemical and vital features and exercise promotes these processes. Diseased areas may be stimulated to a healthy state, circulation may be equalized, innervation may be restored—not by excitement or violence—but by gradual, gentle and harmonious tonic impressions.

Stomach and Digestive Disorders

Included under this general heading are some common chronic disorders of the stomach, with the resulting loss of muscular power and disturbances of the nervous system. The varieties of this disorder are many, and the accompanying symptoms are numerous; but many of them result from the same causes, so very little variation in the treatment is demanded.

The digestion of food may be regarded as a central function upon which the integrity of all other functions is dependent. No function of the body can be properly understood when considered apart from its physiological interrelationships.

Digestion involves the reduction of solid alimentary materials into fluids, able to enter the circulation and supply material for the organizing processes. This act is effected in the digestive cavity formed by the alimentary canal which, with its expansions and convolutions, extends throughout the body, presenting an inner surface of several square feet. Each portion of this canal is adapted to perform some distinct and necessary function in the process and the function is incomplete if any part of the digestive surface is incapable of performing its allotted share.

This change is effected in food by means of secretions poured into the cavity and mingled with the food derived from all parts of the digestive surface. The extent of this surface is increased by certain appendages called glands whose secretions are conducted into the cavity.

The daily amount of secretions for this exclusive purpose is very large and consists of the following substances:

Saliva .... 3.30 lbs.   Pancreatic juice .. .44 lbs.
Gastric juice .... 14.08 lbs.   Intestinal juice ... .44 lbs.
Bile .... 3.30 lbs.

The combined total amounts to more than twenty-one-and-a-half pounds of solvent secretions whose objective is the solution of the two or three pounds of food that is daily required to sustain the functions of the body.

These secretions are derived from the blood, and their quality and adaptation to the purposes for which they are intended, depend upon the quality of that fluid.

In investigating the causes and remedies for indigestion, it is necessary to inquire into the separate influence exerted by the several factors that take part in the act—namely, food, secretions, and those incidental or temporary conditions of the system directly involved in promoting or impairing its health.

The quality of food is a subject that is receiving much attention today. Taste and fashion must come second—the real consideration to be given to any particular material is, can it be readily assimilated and what is its capacity for supporting all the functional operations of the system?

The organic actions of the body have two major objectives: the construction of the instruments of vital action and the maintenance of the vital temperature. To accomplish this there must be a constant supply of materials capable of being organized, instead of those capable of being oxidized. But of all the products of the organic world, whether produced by the plant or derived from the animal, nature divides life sustaining food material in two distinct types. One is the albuminous type, consisting of vegetables and animal aliment, their derivatives fibrin, gluten, casein, etc. and all the saline matters associated with these: all of them contain nitrogen. The other class, of which starch and oil are examples, contains no nitrogen.

A common cause of imperfect digestion is the consumption of improper foods. Since the system is able to dispose of other matters besides food, the distinctive difference between what is and what is not food is apt to be lost sight of, hence the unconscious abuse.

Another source of injury to digestion arises from disregarding the proper relative proportion of the correct elements in the use of food. In this case, while there may be an insufficiency of some of the elements, others are in surplus amount, so that while the system is loaded with materials, organization and nutrition are at a low standard because the necessary elements are not present in sufficient quantity.

The danger to the health arising under this heading comes from two sources: the employment of too much soluble—that is, saccharine —matter and the rejection of the vitally necessary saline constituents, These are apt to be lost by mechanical refining, for most of the saline elements of edible grains exist in the outer or coarser portions.

It is also important that the amount of food taken be relative to the needs of the system; in other words, proportional to the system's power of dissolution in the stomach and intestines and to its power of elimination. If these limits are exceeded, the materials introduced into the digestive cavity are no longer food but a harmful foreign mass, perhaps even poisonous and irritating to the nerves so as to negatively affect the whole system, including the blood.

Secretions constitute the next great factor in the digestive process. It is through these that the solution of food is effected. If these secretions are deficient or inadequate, an imperfect solution of food must result. There can be no proper digestion unless the peculiar chemical affinities of the digestive secretions are able to overpower all other chemical action in the digestive mass.

All the causes listed above have intrinsic and directly injurious tendencies, but there is evidence to indicate that the unpleasant symptoms resulting from indigestion are largely due to disturbances of the nervous system. Stomach irritation is reflected through the nervous system to all the bodily organs and brings about injurious nutritive changes in remote parts of the body. If the ganglionic centers situated near the stomach become inflamed and rendered incapable of performing their duties, a dysfunctioning of the digestion develops that is difficult to cure.

Poor activity of the digestive organs disturbs the digestive process. Proper digestion is not possible while sensations in the stomach are habitually aroused by food—improper in kind or amount—or by stimulating beverages or drugs.

Two symptoms often arise as a result of the conditions just described, aside from the ordinary ones of loss of power, stomach pain, acidity, etc. One is soreness at the pit of the stomach upon deep pressure; the other is a peculiar sensation of buzzing or ringing in the head. There is much evidence that the latter symptom is due to the connection of the nerves of organic life with the cerebrum. The removal of these symptoms is one of the earliest proofs of the restoration of digestive power.

Another cause of indigestion can be a defect in the general vital action of the system. Viewed in reference to the whole system, digestion may be regarded as being dependent upon the general nutritive processes that are constantly active in every portion of the body. The kind of digestive action, as well as the quality of the product, will therefore depend on the degree of perfection with which all the other processes of the system are performed; for each contributes to the replenishing of the blood. An imperfectly constituted blood, loaded with the results of the faulty vital action of the tissues, and returned to the stomach and intestines, is capable of promoting only poor secretions. These irritate, debilitate, and finally make the central organs diseased and sensitive. The amount of digestive secretions poured daily into the digestive cavity, nearly equals that of the whole mass of the blood from which they are derived.

The cause of indigestion is not only confined to improper food; it is also caused by those voluntary habits which are connected with the vital manifestations of the general system. It is to this source that the quality of the digestive fluids is ultimately referable, because they are produced from blood common to all parts and by the vital power belonging to the local organs. Therefore when the energy of the system is low, the digestion is sure to suffer as a direct consequence.

The digestive process depends no less upon how we act, than upon what we eat. No amount of dieting, however correct per se, will be capable of doing more than mask some of the symptoms of indigestion, so long as the movements of the body are insufficient in amount or faulty in kind.

In cases of indigestion arising from this cause, the amount of pain suffered in the region of the stomach gives no true indication of the severity of the disease. The indications of disease afforded through the nerves are very irregular and unreliable and this serves to retard a cure.

The physician whose prescriptions are directed to the mere salving of this kind of patient's present sufferings is not a safe advisor.

To overcome these particular problems, the capacity—not of the stomach only, but of the whole system—to receive food must be considered. The quantity of food taken by the system always depends upon the general habits of the individual, his physical condition at the time, his mental activity, and the exterior and interior environments.

Drugs, even of the mildest kind, are to be avoided in this kind of disease. The temporary relief they sometimes bring is quite certain to be followed by a proportionate impairment of power and the gravest features of the disease are confirmed by an habitual reliance upon such chemicals. Even cases which later recover, in spite of the use of drugs, serve only as dangerous precedents.

Digestive powers are enhanced by vigorous respiratory action—whether induced by exercise or through continued exposure to low temperatures—because it cleanses the blood and enhances the processes of elimination, thus relieving the system of matters that would otherwise contaminate and poison it. The person suffering from indigestion is generally one whose habits of life have been such as to injuriously limit the amount of air respired. Persons who confine themselves to the atmosphere of warm rooms, seldom exposing themselves to currents of cool out-of-door air, find it difficult to avoid digestive disease. Exercise that is well directed has the effect of urging blood to the surface. Free contact with the air, aided by baths, tends to the same result. These means greatly stimulate the respiratory process and at the same time disperse those central congestions which poorly nourish the dyspeptic conditions of the digestive organs.

Exercise contributes more than all other things—drugs included—to the restoration of the dyspeptic individual. However, when nutrition is imperfect the exertion must be proportionally limited. As the muscular power decreases, it becomes necessary to increase the effort of the will in order to accomplish a given effect. This necessitates an injurious expenditure of nervous power and at the same time causes a preponderance of nervous over muscular action, which is fatal to the health. No exercise is proper which does not increase the capacity for exertion. However, this power is not increased but, on the contrary, diminished if constant excessive demands are made upon the nervous system.

Partial exercise, that is, exercise of one portion of the body exclusively, particularly if it is a central portion, as frequently happens in some of the trades and professions, is also detrimental. Such exercise is apt to excite and maintain congestion in those delicate central organs already affected by disease, while it withdraws circulation from the feet and peripheral parts. It is such cases as these that discourage the individual's desire to exercise.

When persons are conscious of this kind of injury, they should not conclude that all exercise is injurious. Even much stronger exercise, if of the right kind and involving parts remote from the root of the disease, may be undertaken with the highest advantage.

All passive exercise, such as riding on horseback, and sailing, is generally very advantageous to aiding digestion. These passive movements remove impediments in the capillary circulation and assist nutrition. Aeration of the blood and absorption are assisted both from the digestive surface and from the system as a whole. In this way all the powers of the body are equalized, and the organic or formative processes are promoted.

Special movements are well adapted to fulfill all indications in this large class of diseases. The prescription should be made so as to affect all parts of the body successively, beginning with the respiratory region and ending with the feet, legs, abdomen, liver, and stomach. This latter organ should, at first, be approached cautiously or left alone entirely. A difficult case of indigestion requires duplicated movements because there is too little strength for the single ones. In addition, duplicate movements lead to greater control over the circulation than do single movements. But single movements are especially useful for the many people who need to guard against the approaches of disease or overcome its milder forms; they are also useful for the after-treatment of a case cured by duplicated movements.

The plan of treatment in this disease does not materially differ from that which is appropriate in pulmonary afflictions. The most important indications in both are to expand the chest, stimulate the circulation in the extremities and peripheral portions of the body, and promote the production of well-vitalized blood in all tissues throughout the body.

Prescriptions to Relieve Digestive Impairment

Movement numbers are given in parenthesis.
1. Weight-held bending (49).
2. Head-support, leg-raising (22).
3. Wing-stride-standing (9).
4. Sitting, trunk-swaying (39).
5. Stride-kneeling, trunk-twisting (46).
6. Sidewise-lying, hips raising (61).
7. Sitting, trunk-twisting (37).
8. Half-lying, abdomen-kneading (65-1).
9. Hanging, holding (75).

After a formula like the above has been used for awhile,

movements that affect the central portions of the body may be used, as follows:

1. Kneeling, arms-stretching (43).
2. Back lying, head and legs raising (62).
3. Half-kneeling, trunk backward bending (48).
4. Sidewise-lying, leg raising (28).
5. Stride kneeling, sidewise swaying (45).
6. Walk-kneeling, trunk twisting (42).
7. Leg forward-raising (19).
8. Double leg-twisting (24).

Incontinence

The bladder lies in the front part of the pelvic cavity. It is in the front of the rectum in the male and in front of the vagina and uterus in the female. The bladder can hold about one pint of urine. The nerves in the autonomic system stimulate the muscles to retain or expel the urine. These muscles do become flaccid with age, but they can often be helped to regain their strength through a deliberate set of exercises as explained here.

STOMACH LIFT—Stand with your knees bent as shown in Figure 18. Breath regularly and more forcibly each time and finally expel all the air from your lungs. Then raise the chest as high as you can and in this way create a vacuum inside your lungs and stomach. Pull hard on the region of the pelvis until you can observe the genitals moving upward. Retain this position for about five seconds then inhale and let the muscles relax.

When you do this exercise concentrate upon the muscles you are strengthening. Repeat this exercise about twelve times each day.

This exercise is also good for treating digestive problems. It is obviously excellent for a flabby stomach; all the muscles of the stomach area will be strengthened. Women may find this exercise especially valuable in restoring a fallen womb.

After doing this exercise for several weeks, increase the retention time to ten or even twenty seconds, but be careful to relax and release the pressure if you feel the slightest strain.

The stomach lift exercise can be done while sitting in a modified yoga position. Sit cross-legged, tailor fashion. Take the left foot and bend it so that the sole is tucked against the upper portion of the right thigh with the left heel near the genitals. Do not sit on the heel. Then bend the right leg so that the right heel is against the pubic bone and the toes of the right foot fit snugly into the crevice formed by the calf and thigh of the left leg. Close your eyes and concentrate upon the muscles to be strengthened. Proceed with the breathing and holding as for the standing position.

The concentration upon the muscles around the triangle of the bladder may be felt in the sphincter muscles at the exit of the colon.

Medical attention is advised if incontinence is not eliminated by these procedures; there remains the possibility that the problem is caused by an infection in the urinary tract. A physican may request permission to grow a culture from a small quantity of urine. The culture will quickly determine if incontinence is a result of an infection.

LYMPHATIC DISORDERS

Diseases of the lymphatic glands manifest themselves in a great variety of symptoms, differing according to constitution and age. In children, it is noted by a peculiar pallor, dullness of complexion, hypertrophied or inflamed mesenteric glands, tumid abdomen, frequent and urgent bowel movements, shrunken limbs, fetid breath, and an indisposition for play. Eruptions of various kinds may occur upon the skin of the face or other parts of the body, swellings upon or about the neck often appear. The child often presents a haggard, almost wild, appearance and blue veins are painfully prominent.

In adolescence, the most striking symptoms of the affliction are enlarged glands of the neck, fragility of form, narrowness of the chest, a strong tendency to cough, and lung disease which frequently develops into pulmonary consumption.

In adults, the disease is apt to center in the lungs. There is a period when sufficient knowledge and a correct practice would effectively bar the progress of the disease. We ought to seek the preventive rather than the curative practice since prevention is possible.

In this disease, the results of the vital processes are incompletely attained. The mesenteric glands and the lymphatic vessels become clogged with the materials of an imperfect nutrition, while the skin and lungs execute their functions in an unsatisfactory manner. The result is either that the nutritive elements become imperfectly vitalized, or that matters destined to be eliminated as waste from the system fail to become converted into the usual soluble forms of carbonic acid, water, and urea. Hence occur the excess of albuminous material and the imperfect and irregular cells that characterize the scrofulous deposits of the lungs, glandular system, etc., The nature of the mischievous agents that work together in the production of these conditions is learned by a study of the disease during its development and subsequent progress.

Among the prominent causes of this disease are insufficiency of pure air, light, and exercise, and want of cleanliness. We have only to look into the abodes of poverty and squalor for confirmation of this statement.

But even those living in wealthier environments are apt to be afflicted with lymphatic diseases and, oddly, for much the same reasons as the poor. In both cases respiration is rendered ineffectual by circumstances that are somehow similiar. There is a lack of healthful motion and purity of air, and these effects are aggravated by want of exercise and good habits on the part of the persons thus exposed. It is not the uncleanliness external to the body that exercises the most deleterious influence upon the health. It is when matters foreign to the purposes of the body become constituents of its substances, that the most serious interference with the vital operations occurs. The liability of being poisoned through the lungs is immeasurably greater than of being poisoned through the skin. No amount of washing and bathing are effectual if other habits preclude a free access of air to the skin and lungs. There are no hygienic or medical procedures which can possibly compensate for this need.

Heredity may influence this form of disease because the original form of the body is inherited: the narrow chest of the lymphatically diseased child is inherited along with the color of his eyes and the contour of his face. But the practice of exercise therapy can modify the shape and size of the members and regions of the body.

Exercise-therapy secures a greater degree of energy in all the formative or organic actions of the system, especially those agencies which favor the oxidizing processes in the blood and solid tissues such as light, exercise, and wholesome and invigorating food. Through the assimilation of drugs the disease may be masked and so seemingly improved, but the results are temporary and uncertain.

Exercise therapy gives direction and energy to the vitalizing processes throughout the body, and causes a renewal of the fluids of the clogged glandular system, relieves glandular congestion, and supplies oxygen to impoverished blood. In this way the non-vitalized and imperfectly vitalized matters of the blood, and of the body are reduced, the chest is enlarged, and the power of the system to continue its numerous operations in a healthful manner is maintained and augmented.

The person with this type of disease needs every available hygienic resource. He cannot effectually combat the advancing disease simply by attending to one or two particulars of remedial hygiene. He should abstain from all drugs, condiments, strong beverages, stimulants, etc., and should adhere to a simple nutritious diet, selecting foods that possess the particular elements he needs. He must not compel his digestive apparatus to reduce needless matter to the necessary forms in which they may exit from the body, for all such matter require the oxygen that might and ought to be employed in eliminating the disease.

The body's strength, in these cases, is generally already impaired and the patient, consequently, should avoid such exercises as might tend to exhaust the physical powers.

In this disease, the functioning of the breathing organs is diminished and becomes an impediment to recovery. The deficiency in dimensions may be either congenital or acquired. In either case it is receptive to therapy and it should be one of the first objectives of treatment.

The circumference of the chest and waist may be astonishingly increased by proper exercise and nutritive measures, and the several cubic inches of increased capacity that is afforded to the lungs increases the respiratory ability in a commensurate degree. A change for the better in health is almost immediate. Food is not only reduced to fluidity and enabled to pass the digestive elements into the blood, but becomes transformed into a healthy vital element instead of remaining in organic form and becoming an obstruction to the healthy growth of the system. A higher vital tone and energy is thus secured, and good health is the natural consequence.

Duplicated movements are demanded if the case is a formidable one, and these should be continued for several weeks, or until evidence of improvement becomes apparent. Later, if the illness is not too severe, the single movements may be employed with benefit.

The movements prescribed for this patient should be similiar to those recommended for pulmonary afflictions, but they may, from the first, be used more energetically. All portions of the body should be included in the movements, so that all the organs and functions of the system may share the effect. But the special indication, or indications, of the case should be emphasized. If there is a tendency of blood to flow to the head excessively, the prescription should begin with movements of the lower extremities and afterward move to the arms and chest. If there is constipation, movements adapted to this particular complaint should be included. If there are no special indications, the prescription should begin with movements for the chest.

Prescriptions for Lymphatic Disorders

The following movements will serve as examples:

1. Foot-rotation (passive) (7).
2. Sitting, arm twisting (71).
3. Trunk rotation (74).
4. Stride-kneeling, sidewise swaying (45).
5. Kneeling, knee-stretching (12).
6. Half-standing, leg rotation (23).
7. Sitting, trunk twisting (37).
8. Stretch backward-lying (67).

Movement numbers are in parentheses.

MOTOR PARALYSIS

Exercise therapy offers hope to this obstinate affliction. Other remedies, such as strychnine, stimulants, galvanism, or electricity, may afford relief by their temporary effects, and so they may seem to do a great deal of good. But they only exhaust the recuperative powers, and the case can only become less amenable to proper treatment.

The treatment of paralysis by duplicated movements has resulted in favorable improvements. Patients with useless and burdensome limbs have had their power partially or even entirely restored. Patients who have been completely paraplegic for several years have been restored to health and the active pursuit of their professions.

Sometimes the cause of paralysis is some defect in the nerve centers located in the spinal cord and at the base of the brain. From these the incentive to muscular action originates. These centers consist of the grey substance of the cord, and they communicate by means of countless radiating nerve fibers connected to all the muscular tissue of the body.

The actual pathological state of these nerve centers in paralysis is often an obscure matter. It may be that the walls of the capillary vessels supplying the part with nutrition have ruptured, and effusion of a clot, pressure, and a sudden shock, deprives the parts or muscles connected therewith by the nerve fibers. The extent of the paralysis will depend on the location. Those portions of the body connected with the cord below the seat of disease will suffer from its effect.

Another cause may be serious effusion into the membrane enclosing the cord which may, by its pressure, gradually produce similar symptoms.

Sometimes a disease of the substance of the cord occurs, called softening, and destroys the function of the cord and of the parts connected with it. The muscles are not primarily affected but their action, becoming suspended, is deprived of nutrition. Consequently they become weak, flabby, and diminished. The nerve filaments which conduct the nerve influence from its central seat aren't necessarily implicated. They cease to conduct impressions simply because they receive none in the disabled state of the central organ.

The reader may wonder how exercise of the muscles which are not at the seat of the disease can restore functional power to the disabled nerve.

The spinal column is enclosed in the bony case formed by the vertebral column which protects it from injury from external sources, and is suspended and surrounded through its entire length by fluid. By this arrangement, injury to the cord from any sudden twist or shock is usually prevented.

But this is not all. Along the exterior surface of the column is situated the largest and strongest muscular mass belonging to the body, which is employed in sustaining and giving flexibility and mobility to the trunk. Every action of these muscles necessarily affects the circulation of the contained and contiguous vessels, and modifies the condition of the contents of the vertebral canal. The lateral forward, backward, and diagonal inclinations of the body in the duplicated and single movements are eminently derivative for the cord itself and serve as a powerful means for relieving congestion of the spinal membranes and nerves, or even for removing serious effusion.

In many cases, the spinal lesion has recovered spontaneously. Still, the power of motion is not, as a consequence, restored.

The paralysis generally continues because the conductor, having ceased to perform its duty, continues inoperative even after the original source of nerve power is restored by time. It is evident that the muscles will remain inactive so long as the nerves refuse to convey motive force to them. It is inferred that this state of things may often exist for the simple reason that very frequently paralysis is speedily overcome by movements; this could not happen if the cord itself, the source of all muscular power, remained diseased. The cure, in this case, does not consist of the removal of disease, but in the restoration of a function. The germ of the power to move still exists; this is to be encouraged and cultivated. The disabled muscles must be moved, and helped to move themselves, until they have regained the ability to work unassisted.

Exercise therapy often overcomes this formidable disease by removing any pressure that may exist at the nerve centers and by restoring the flow of nervous force to its original channels. At the same time, the general expenditure of nerve power is carefully secured by tranquilizing the whole system, especially the diseased organs, and by re-establishing the conditions for healthy nutrition throughout the body. Exercise therapy depreciates the employment of any means designed merely to stimulate the nerves to functional activity. It rejects all beverages except simple unadulterated water. The use of tobacco may aggrevate the disease, as might the use of spicey food of all kinds, which never replenish nerve power. For the same reason, exercise therapy enjoins abstinence from everything calculated to arouse the emotions or awaken anxious or laborious thought, for these things tend to debilitate the nervous system, and must necessarily aggravate the disease, counteracting the beneficial effects of the therapy.

Prescriptions for Motor Paralysis

The prescription must embrace bending, falling, etc., for such positions call the muscles of the back, and especially the neck, into active play. It should include attempts at the restoration of power in the defective members. The liver should be aroused into activity by regulating and restricting the diet and by employing the appropriate movements. Many of the duplicated movements of the passive kind are important here for the toning up of defective nerves and those organs whose actions are limited through lack of nervous supply, as well as to soothe and tranquilize the nerves themselves. Such movements are to be applied very cautiously in the vicinity of nerve centers, more freely along the conductors.

It is important to direct the attention of the nerve force into the affected part by attempting to move the debilated or disabled part and the power must be applied by an assistant. Unless the patient eventually sees improvement accomplished by his own endeavors, he will be disheartened and give up his efforts. If the paralytic cannot raise his hands he must at least try. The patient does not know that he exerts any power until he has exerted enough to accomplish his purpose. If he is assisted he can be made to feel that he overcomes a part of the resistance and thus be encouraged to continue and multiply his efforts.

All of the patient's motions should be deliberate and gentle. The time of the movement should not be prolonged and the part moved should be sustained during a period of rest at the terminal position. In this way the objective of the movement, which consists of establishing and improving the communication between the nerve centers and muscles, is secured as much as possible. It is only necessary to repeat the same movement at the same time, and in the same way daily, and an increased—if not a perfect—control of the weakened part is quite certain to result. But if, on the other hand, the movements be taken at irregular times and practiced rapidly, violently, or carelessly, energy will be exhausted rather than increased, and injury will result.

CONSTIPATION

Among those people engaged in sedentary lifestyles, no condition is more common than constipation of the bowels and none is more disregarded. Often constipation is the first notice given of the beginning of a state of chronic ill health that can prove permanent. This problem may exist even when the individual is not aware of the fact; for though his evacuations may be regular, the residual matter occupies a much longer time in its passage through the canal than is compatible with health.

The symptom is often accompanied by disorder of the stomach, and is frequently connected with nervous irritability, prostration, hypochondria, etc. It is apt to accompany the first stages of pulmonary disease and, indeed, nearly all persons afflicted with chronic disorders are troubled with costiveness.

Prominent among the causes of this condition are sedentary habits, anxiety of mind and severe thinking, a prolonged use of improper foods, and the indulgence of aperients (laxatives) and other drugs. Constipation may be connected with other symptoms which constitute the main disease, but generally it is the result of one, or of a combination of the causes mentioned. Persons of active lifestyles who do not unduly burden themselves with cares and anxieties, are not apt to be afflicted in this manner.

Improper food poisons rather than nourishes the body; it induces congestion of the alimentary canal by the irritation it sets up and by the effects of the chemical changes it undergoes in that canal. Cathartic drugs are foreign to body needs, wear down the delicate vital susceptibility, and aggravate the disease for which they are applied. The relief they afford is transitory and deceitful.

Under the combined influence of improper habits and

laxatives, the afflicted individual is apt to go from bad to worse. Many persons are slaves to the enema, the only substitute they know for the pills or bolus. This is perhaps a less harmful remedy, but it is still unsatisfactory. We can not really cure the disease which causes retention of fecal matter while we confound this symptom with the disease itself.

We must look to the causes of constipation from several distinct viewpoints, then we shall be able to remove them.

1. A weakness of the muscular covering of the alimentary canal exists, so that its vermicular and expulsive power becomes insufficient.

2. There is a defect in the power of the lower section of the spinal cord. The defective power of the expulsive muscles, especially those of the inferior portion of the tube, results partly from a lack of nervous power. This is the natural consequence of the energy being too largely drawn from improper areas such as the brain and the stomach. It is necessary to stop this improper energy drain and to use appropriate means to stimulate the nervous power in the part of the body where it is especially needed. The lower section of the cord should be roused to action chiefly by means of the muscles supplied from this source—occasionally by more direct operations.

3. There may exist congestion of the mucous membrane of some part of the alimentary tube which causes a deficiency of the required secretions. This state of the mucous membranes calls for the exercise and development of the abdominal coverings for the purpose of drawing off the blood from the congested parts into the acting

ones, thus relieving that state. Motion applied to the membrane—or rather to the organs of which the membrane is a part—is also needed to assist the capillary action in the membrane.

4. The abdominal muscles whose function it is to assist the expulsive efforts are, in constipation, flabby, doughy and weak. They fail both to maintain the abdominal contents in the proper situation and to act with sufficient force to aid materially in the contraction of the tube. This state may be readily remedied by the exercises.

5. The liver is apt to be torpid and congested. Sometimes this state is indicated by tenderness in the region of this organ. This condition manifests imperfect oxidation of the blood and a retention of matters that ought to have been reduced through respiration to a soluble form and expelled from the body. These retained matters are proximate elements of the bile. The tissues are wanting in moisture because the refuse materials of the system are not throughly reduced as they should be, to carbonic acid and water. To remedy this case, movements to improve respiratory action are demanded, together with a reduction in the amount of food consumed. In this way the harmonious co-operation of the digestive and respiratory functions are restored.

6. Circulation is poor and blood collects in excess in the large central vessels, robbing the extremities of their proper supply. Cold hands and feet are a symptom of this particular form. Movements prescribed for the extremities—which will draw the blood toward them—are necessary to effect a wholesome distribution of the circulation.

Consider, by contrast, the modus operandi of laxatives:

1. The drug being mixed with the homogeneous contents of the intestinal tube and impregnating the whole of the contained mass, is incongruous to the purpose for which nutritive matters are designed; the absorbents, therefore, refuse to take up matters thus contaminated. Hence nutrition is suspended and there is, for a time, a general decline in strength.

2. The mass, now having become offensive to the organic instinct, is acted upon by the emunctories with great power in order to free the system from impending harm. By this means the whole intestinal mass, rendered partly fluid by imperfect digestion, is forced rapidly through the entire length of the tube.

3. Some portions of the offensive matter are absorbed into the blood but are then directly returned to the intestinal canal as being the appropiate way of exiting the body. This portion is mingled with serum drawn from the blood, so as to dilute the noxious principle and thus prevent, to a degree, the injury resulting from its immediate contact with vital parts.

4. In the operations just described, only one advantage has been gained and this is incidental and indirect. While nutrition is prevented from entering the blood, respiration continues as usual. The poisonous matters which are prone to become destructive have been reduced in the ordinary way, and have made their exit from the system rapidly.

The effects produced by cathartics are the same and are more quickly and easily obtained. However, in the cathartic process the true cause of constipation is not addressed and it continues to exist after the operation of the medicine. The system has been relieved only for the moment while the disease, thus masked, has acquired fresh power.

The cure for constipation can lie in movements. If the case is of great severity, the duplicated movements are called for; but the single movements are competent to subdue minor complaints.

Prescriptions for Constipation

The following prescriptions for movements will be found to be powerfully remedial in an ordinary case of constipation. Movement numbers are given in parenthesis.

1. Wing-stride-standing (9).
2. Trunk vibration (64).
3. Thigh-rotation (31).
4. Lying, legs-rotation (29).
5. Sidewise-lying, hips raising (61).
6. Stride-kneeling, sidewise swaying (45).
7. Head-support, leg raising (22).
8. Abdominal kneading (65-1).
9. Spine knocking (32).
10. Long-sitting, trunk forward bending (53).
11. Leg stretching (16).
12. Legs-separation (27).

All the above movements affect the abdominal and

pelvic contents. There are several others which act more remotely upon the same parts. In making a formula of treatment, some three or four of the above movements may be selected and these should be used in conjunction with derivative movements for the feet and hands, as suited to the strength of the patient.

EXAMPLE 1.

These movements may be repeated as necessary. In addition to this treatment, an enema of tepid water may be employed from time to time although its habitual use should be avoided. A tepid hip-bath may also be used occasionally if found to be agreeable to the patient. But it is futile to employ exercise to restore the health of the digestive organs while ignoring the general lifestyle that contributes to the affliction.

CHRONIC DIARRHEA AND COLITIS

Several causes may underlie this symptom, and they may act either singly or concurrently.

1. General relaxation of the tissues, or debility, is always present and refers to some imperfection of the primary actions.

2. The presence of crude and irritating matters in the alimentary canal causes spasmodic action of the muscular covering while at the same time absorption of the contents is prevented by the diseased state of the membrane. The alimentary mass is consequently rapidly dismissed.

3. In case of sudden poisoning of the blood—either

from spontaneous metamorphosis, as in cholera, or the accidental or prescribed use of some injurious drug—the alimentary canal furnishes a ready outlet so that destructive matters may be eliminated. In this instance, diarrhea is a curative action on the part of nature and the symptoms generally amount to something more than is generally understood by the term diarrhea.

4. An ulcerated patch (colitis) may exist in the canal, causing diarrhea.

5. The relaxation of the abdominal parietes and contents, and the consequent pressure upon the perineum and sphincter muscles, may excite action of the lower bowel. This results in a strong urge and much straining—a reflexive nervous effect of pressure upon the sphincter. In this case there is prolapsus of the bowels, either concealed or apparent.

In each of the above cases, except where the action is acute, what is needed is improved muscle tone of the vital structure. The vital organization is depressed and incomplete and the true remedy must be something that will restore power and activity. The fluids of the system must be conveyed from the digestive center outward to the remote parts of the body. The arterial action is low and needs to be energized; there is venous plethora and poor respiration. The muscular tissue is lax and weak and all the organizing processes of the body are carried on slowly and unsteadily. These difficulties are often overcome by the application of the healing movements.

At first the movements prescribed should be of the passive sort. For this reason all vibratory movements applied to the abdomen produce good effects, their extent corresponding to the thoroughness and faithfulness with which they are applied. One may vibrate and knead his own abdomen in any of several ways with much benefit. At the same time, it is useful to apply movements to the extremities for the purpose of drawing the blood away from the central organs and also to promote the respiratory process in order to restore the purity of this fluid. In the case of ulceration of the bowels, long, persistent, and careful constitutional treatments are required. Short, cold sitting-baths aid the respiration and encourage the contractile efforts of the bowels.

HEMORRHOIDS

This affliction often consists of a distention of the veins at the posterior termination of the mucous lining of the intestine. It is accompanied by a sensitiveness caused by a sluggishness of the abdominal circulation and, generally, an engorgement of the liver may be presumed. The condition of the liver is such as to retard the flow of blood in the portal veins which return the blood to the heart from the region of the digestive tube. Hence, the lower branches of the veins that contribute to the portal circulation become distended. Inflammation follows the distention of the hemorrhoidal veins, and they often become hardened, ulcerated and disposed to bleed easily. Sometimes a considerable loss of blood occurs from this state.

Sometimes there is a prolapsus of the rectum, which greatly aggravates the disorder, as a result of the constant straining efforts made in evacuating the bowels. This retards the upward flow and the vessels of the sphincter become strangulated.

The treatment is used, first, to relieve the liver of congestion and reduce the abdominal plethora by temporarily eliminating the intake of solid foods. This aids the contraction of the surcharged vessels and also removes the impediment to the onward flow of the blood. Secondly, it aims to draw the abdominal contents upward and relieve the pressure upon the sphincter. Thirdly, it must remove the capillary congestion of the parts.

Surgical intervention may be indicated in severe cases of this disease.

In lieu of the duplicated movements, single movements may be employed for this affliction to great advantage. The objective should be to affect the liver and arouse the abdominal circulation to greater activity. The following exercises are suggested:

1. Elbows support lying (76).
2. Rack grasp, forward falling (68).
3. Stretch backward-lying (67).

DEFORMITIES OF THE SPINE

The application of proper exercises to the correction of spinal curvatures is especially successful and satisfying. Not only is relief obtained but there is also a visual benefit.

In order to arrive at some conclusions about exercise

treatment it is necessary to inquire about the origin of the spinal deformity. The anatomical character and relations of the column itself and of its supports must be considered. The column consists of twenty-four light, spongy bones, resting their flat surfaces upon each other, with a cushion of elastic cartilage between. This interposition of cartilage is necessary for flexibility and elasticity in resisting the shocks to which the spine is so often subjected. It also gives the trunk the pliability and freedom of motion necessary in daily life.

The form and construction of the spinal column could not possibly maintain an erect position without the control of muscles which are attached to it at many points and are capable of supporting it in every direction and position. The muscular connections of the spinal column with other parts of the body are extensive and various. The arms and legs are connected to it by muscles, and consequently the character of their motions is related to the positions of the spine. Conversely, the movements of these members are, to a considerable extent, capable of modifying its form.

The spinal column, in its normal condition, is far from straight. It has several curves: forward at the neck, and lumbar region and backward in its dorsal section, and at the loins. These curves increase the elasticity of the column and are necessary to the symmetry of the body, favoring the natural action of the muscles,

The spine can be incorrectly curved in two ways: vertically and laterally. Natural curves are vertical, front to back; if these curves are excessive, the body's shape is deformed by exaggeration. This kind of curvature occurs because the muscles which should hold the spine straighter are weak. As a result, the weight of the body is badly supported and the supple column yields at its weakest point—the extremity of the curve.

The second form of curvature is lateral; that is, viewed from the back, the spine is curved sideways, instead of being straight. This is the result of weakness in muscles which control the movement and general position of the trunk.

Lateral curvatures form a group for which movements furnish a satisfactory remedy.

Lateral curvatures may be single or double. In the former case the middle portion of the spinal column deviates, causing one portion of the body to form a more convex line than the other. In the latter case the shape of the column somewhat resembles the italic S. In the greater number of cases there is more upper deviation to the right, and more lower spine deviation to the left.

There is also a twisting of the trunk: one shoulder projects forward, twisting the chest and pelvis in an abnormal way.

Spinal deformities assume many different shapes, no two are exactly alike. They all require a competent physician for diagnosis and proper prescription. The greater frequency of right-lateral curvatures is evidently connected with the greater use, and consequently power, of the right arm and muscles of the right side: this causes the dorsal vertebrae to be drawn with greater frequency and force in that direction.

Curvatures to the right consequently cause greater development of the right than of the left arm. There

exists in most persons the same greater proportional use
of the right leg as of the right arm. One leads with the
right leg oftener, and more frequently rests upon it, than
the left. While one is thus resting upon a single leg, the
horizontal plane of the pelvis is caused to incline toward
the side imperfectly supported. Consequently, the spinal
column is no longer straight as it should be but becomes
bent toward the right single side. Since this deviation
of the spine would cause the body to fall, it compensates
and curves in the opposite direction at a lower place on
the spinal column.

The lateral curvature of the spine is the product of one
of two causes. The weakness of the muscles is so great
as to leave the column unsupported, in which case it
yields to the weight of the superior portion of the body.
Or the greater use and development of one side of the
body interferes with the harmonious action of the opposing muscles of the two sides. In either case a change
in the shape of the bones must ultimately take place,
and a deformity occurs, with impairment. The character
of the deformity varies. It may be modified by a variety
of circumstances such as the influence of particular habits
and postures: a habit of reclining mostly on one side, of
studying, writing, or other occupations that employ
chiefly one or the other side of the body, whether in the
sitting or standing posture; and it may even follow as the
effect of diseases of the internal organs.

Curvature of the spine may also result from predisposition to lymphatic disease. In this case ulcerative absorption of some portion of the vertebral column takes
place, most commonly at the front in the dorsal region

where the inner edges of the contiguous vertebrae are subject to the most pressure. The effect of this is to cause the vertebra within which this process is going on to acquire more of a wedge shape; the inner edge of the bone is worn away, allowing the column to bend at this point and producing an unsightly prominence or angle. In this case, the cartilage being removed, the bones become irremediably united or, technically speaking, anchylosed.

In the above cases, as long as the causes continue, the deformity has a tendency to increase, and eventually become extremely injurious to the health. The internal organs may become displaced, so as to prevent the performance of their functions; or the spinal cord may become compressed, producing neuralgia or partial paralysis of the lower extremities. No remedies supplied through the stomach are helpful and, generally, the only recourse of the physician has been artificial supports and mechanical extension.

The result of this kind of treatment is not satisfactory. The reason is apparent. The mechanical support affords relief to the fatigued parts and removes the painful pressure on one side. But this is an effectual barrier to the nutrition and development of the natural muscular supports. Consequently, their condition, instead of improving, is certain to grow worse. Thus the disease and accompanying deformity, instead of being removed, are perpetuated. The great majority of the spinal supporters are contrived to take the place of the muscles and to do their duty, which is an impossibility, and their influence is consequently harmful. They subject the chronically sickly child or adolescent to a torture that is not only unnecessary, but is also injurious to the general health.

Spinal deformities are the result of muscular weakness, which is the product of imperfect muscular nutrition, often referable defective digestion. The trouble is often aggravated, and in some cases induced, by irregular innervation, producing spasm of certain muscles. In ordinary cases the therapeutic indications are simple, plain, and unequivocal, and consist in developing the power of the digestive and muscular system, thus enabling the latter to do the duties it has failed to perform. The means for effecting these goals do not reside with any medications to be swallowed at certain times of the day and night, nor with mechanical supports and complex modes of extensions, but simply in the practice of movements, which are the only proper and efficient means of calling the needed nutrition into the disabled parts, so as to reinstate them to health and power.

In directing the treatment of deformities by single movements, it is only necessary that the movements be directed exclusively to the development of the weaker parts. For instance, in right lateral curvature, the movements should be directed to the left side, and in the ordinary exercises of the invalid the left side should always have the preference, while much exertion of the muscles of the right should, for a while, be avoided. If serious attention is paid to this, the nutrition of the two sides of the body will soon be equalized and their muscular forces balanced.

It is not difficult by means of duplicated and single movements to improve the shape of the spinal column

and—if the vertebrae are in sound condition—the restoration of symmetry will be complete. But if the vertebrae have become considerably diseased and misshapen,
the degree of improvement attained will be less. In such
cases judicious mechanical aid is useful, but this must
not be at the expense of the muscles. This assistance
should be directed solely to the rectification of the shape
of vertebral bones and consist of simply applying pressure to the projecting point, wherever that may be. This
is accomplished by means of ingeniously contrived instruments, nicely adapted to the purpose. But these aids
are never used except in conjunction with appropiate
and vigorously applied movements, for without these,
the artificial appliances are useless, if not harmful.

Prescriptions for Spinal Curvature

In a case of simple curvature to the right, the invalid
may employ the following movements with great advantage:

1. Hanging (left arm) (75).
2. Knee bending (left leg) (10).
3. Step standing, trunk bending to the right (four times)
    (51).
4. Trunk bending to the right (36).
5. Short-sitting, forward falling leftward (33).

19   Female Diseases

Many women suffer from diseases peculiar to their sex. The most common problems to be solved are the troublesome ones of: premenstrual distress, bladder infections, urinary control problems, dysmenorrhea and menopausal suffering.

The symptoms that attend this class of diseases include a laxity of muscular fiber. This is manifested even in facial expressions and the way one walks. There is apt to be an inability to walk any considerable distance without fatigue, which is generally felt in the back and loins, and thence down to the limbs. Back pain is apt to be very persistent. The act of ascending stairs may be laborious and difficult, followed by an aggravation of distressing symptoms. There is apt to be a tenderness of the lower portion of the abdomen, accompanied by a dragging sensation, pain, urinary derangement, and sensitiveness of the lower extremity of the spinal column, followed by headache and other symptoms, both local and general.

Sustaining the body with mechanical supporters is destructive to the health of the muscles, and hence to that of the general system. The use of supports distends and irritates the parts and disturbs their natural functions.

Stimulants and tonic drugs are often employed; these temporarily deceive the patient but their ultimate effect impairs the assimilative and vital power. Prescribing inactivity or suspension of the natural functions, although they would be the best condition for recruiting strength, is also common.

These means alternately tantalize and depress the sufferer with hopes and fears, and prevent both patient and medical advisor from attending to the real fundamental causes of the misery and from the employment of the appropiate means for its relief.

The existence of the above symptoms doesn't always indicate the existence of local congestion or of local disease. There may be organic disease. Even when there is ulceration of the neck of the uterus, hypertrophy of that organ, leucorrhea, etc., the gravity of the case does not reside in these symptoms, but in the lack of vital energy which permits these symptoms to occur. The common medical practice allows these signs to continually recur. No reliable permanent cure can be effected while the disease is regarded as residing in the symptoms, which should be considered as only proofs of its existence.

The real pathology of these diseases consists in such conditions as defective muscular nutrition and tone, defective peripheral circulation, central congestion, defective innervation, heightened nervous susceptibility, and bad digestion—the latter three conditions depending on the first three.

The causes of the disease lie in a culture that often ignores the physiological needs of the female body.

The exterior shape conveys but a slight idea of the muscular weakness for there are a number of other muscles, beyond the reach of direct observation, which are equally important to the health of these parts—such as the internal muscles of locomotion, the rotary muscles of the thigh, and especially those of the floor of the pelvis.

The health of the pelvic organs is dependent, as are those of the abdominal, upon the oscillatory motion communicated by the diaphragm in respiration. A decrease of this motion favors congestion in the capillary circulation of those organs which have but little independent motion and tend to rely on that received from neighboring muscles.

The health of the pelvic organs is very much contingent upon the mechanical effects produced upon them by respiration. But the health of the chest and that of the abdomen are associated in another manner. With distention of the lower portion of the abdominal walls its contents sink and the diaphragm, which is the superior boundary of the abdominal cavity, must also descend. The ribs necessarily become depressed, the cavity of the chest becomes narrowed, and the breathing capacity is consequently diminished.

The proper digestion of food and healthful blood are also dependent on vigorous respiration. Now, at the bottom of many female problems lies the faulty condition of the blood. But poor blood does a worse thing than produce weakness; it creates congestion, and the most dependent organs, especially those with no voluntary muscular contractility, such as the uterus, are most likely to suffer. The peculiar congestion preceding and accompanying the menstrual flow may become chronic because of inadequate operation of the muscles and add to the trouble. When we consider the universality of these causes, we wonder that so many women manage to escape these difficulties.

The remedy suited to this large and distressing class of complaints is suggested by their pathology. In cases of displacement of various kinds; congestion, ulceration, etc., of the womb, and afflictions of other organs associated with it, such as the bladder and ovaries, the treatment by exercise has proven more beneficial than either surgical or medical remedies. Through movement, the organs may be raised to their normal positions and retained there because of their own restored power. By means of the most simple instruction in the principles and practice of movements, the condition of the health of the region in question is placed under the control of the patient.

Treatment in these cases is as follows:

1. To elevate the ribs and diaphragm and increase the space of the superior portion of the abdominal cavity.

2. To contract the space of the inferior portion of the same cavity by causing a permanent contraction of the muscular walls of this region.

3. To develop the small muscles about the thighs and those constituting the floor of the pelvis.

4. To remove the blood from the weak and therefore congested internal parts to peripheral parts, abdominal coverings, and extremities.

5. To restore health to the mental and nervous systems by diminishing nervous irritability.

6. To impart vital energy that shall be radical and permanent to the whole system.

The particular movements required to fulfill these indications depend upon the temperament and the health of the patient. If there is a great weakness, the duplicated movements are indispensible to the successful treatment and should be employed at the beginning. If there is much tenderness of the abdomen, then vibratory and other passive movements for the central portions of the body can be interspersed with more active ones. After a few days the extremities will be better supplied with blood and the visceral congestion will be diminished so that pressures, bendings, etc., will be easily executed and gratifying to the patient. After this is accomplished, the patient may carry on the cure alone. If the disease is not far advanced, treatment can begin with the single movements.

Prescriptive Movements

Movement numbers appear in parentheses.
1. Stretch backward-lying (67).
2. Elbows-and-toes lying (60).
3. Trunk lying, leg raising (26).
4. Thigh rotation (31).
5. Reclining, knee-stretching (30).
   Repeat—
1. Kneeling, arm stretching (43).

2. Long-sitting, trunk forward-bending (53).
3. Short-sitting, backward-falling (34).
4. Head-support, leg raising (22).
5. Spine knocking (32).
6. Double leg-twisting (24).
7. Sidewise-lying, hips raising (61).
8. Leg stretching (16).
9. Lying, legs-rotation (29).
10. Feet rotation (5).

In selecting movements for these afflictions, the nature of each case must be carefully considered. Generally, appropriate movements should be applied to the extremities at first. The more diseased the case, the fewer movements directly affecting the central organs should be employed. The movement should be taken once a day, and if there is sufficient ability, number two of the first group, or numbers one or three of the second, may be repeated, according to the mode described, several times in the course of the day.

If the patient has a tilting forward (anteversion) or backward (retroversion) of the uterus, or other serious displacements, her movements should be prescribed by a competent physician.

By following these rules, the women afflicted with these female disorders will, in a few weeks, find their strength greatly improved. They will feel the influx of health in their bodies.

However, two other female problems helped by movement therapy are:

PROLAPSUS OF THE WOMB AND BOWELS—In most cases of this kind there is a great weakness of the muscles of the chest, abdomen, perineum, etc. To strengthen the parts that are weak and prevent a relapse, the muscles belonging to all the above mentioned regions require development by judicious practice of the exercises affecting such movements.

AMENORRHEA—All processes tending to strengthen the body also tend to overcome menstrual obstruction. Movements are particularly recommended as therapeutic aid in relieving congestion and pelvic distress.

The following movements are useful, with movement numbers given in parentheses.
1. Wing stride-standing (9).
2. Knee bending (10).
3. Head-support, leg-raising (22).
4. Half-standing, leg rotation (23).
5. Leg sideways-raising (21).
6. Trunk lying, leg raising (26).
7. Lying, legs rotation (29).
8. Spine knocking (32).

Movement numbers 14, 18, 27, 30, and 31 are also helpful for this condition, as are the foot movements generally.

The auxiliary means are important here. The patient must observe a proper and healthful diet and avoid highly seasoned food, stimulants, and all indigestible matters. She must obtain adequate vitamins and nutrients needed to correct faulty nuitrition and inadequate glandular activity.

20 Miscellaneous Ailments and Movements

Chronic Fatigue

It is not necessary to abstain from motion altogether in order to secure rest from fatigue. On the contrary, the continuance of exercise may be more favorable to restoration than a state of total inactivity, provided that the fatigued parts are not called into action. This is the advantage of a change of occupation, especially for the weak. One can accomplish a great deal more in a given time by varying the work occasionally, than by expending strength upon only one kind. All animals instinctively stretch themselves, or otherwise cause the muscles situated remotely from the central organs to act, in order to get relief from the sense of fatigue.

Exercise therapy regards the body as a reservoir of force upon which every action makes a certain demand. If the demands upon the system are moderate, the supply is readily kept equal to the demand by the unceasing operations of the organizing processes. If the demand is excessive and the organizing processes are not equal to it, fatigue is the consequence. Immunity from fatigue is experienced in proportion to the degree of perfection attained by the nutritive or organizing processes.

It must not be inferred that exercise is always the appropiate remedy for fatigue. If the fatigue is general, absolute rest is necessary.

Nose-Bleed

Raise both arms to the upward stretch position. The efficacy for this action is simple. If the arms are raised to the perpendicular upright position and then, after remaining uplifted for a short time, permitted suddenly to drop, the hands will be suffused with blood. Since a much greater impediment than usual is presented to flow of blood by the uplifted hands and the force of gravity, the effort of the arterial vessels becomes necessarily much greater than before. And since the arterial pressure in direction of the arms is increased, that toward the head is correspondingly lessened. The blood, now rushing to the hands, produces a marked derivative effect upon the circulation to the head, and consequently the flow from the ruptured capillaries of the nasal membranes ceases.

Chronic Headache

1. Energetic friction applied over the longitudinal, lateral, and basilar sinuses will frequently relieve this

affliction. The reason seems to be that contraction is thus induced in the venous walls and urges the blood forward, relieving the walls of their distention. This may be done by oneself, or by another. The procedure is as follows: partly close the hands, placing the backs of the fingers in contact, raise the hands to the head, placing the tips of all the fingers over the longitudinal suture, or middle of the head. Now carry the fingers, thus placed, backward and forward on the middle line, making considerable friction upon the scalp. The fingers may now divide and pass down the back of the head at each side to the base, and then along the base at the roots of the hair, continuing the same degree of friction through the whole course.

2. If a band is very tightly applied about the head and, after remaining a few minutes, is suddenly removed, a similiar effect is experienced.

3. Movements tending to warm the feet are always useful in headaches. In moderate cases, a long walk in the open air is sufficient. If this is not enough, abstinence must be practiced till the stomach is clear, the liver relieved of the tenderness and congestion that may exist, and the secretions set free. Nervous headaches require rest and sleep and/or the release obtained through meditation.

Hernia

This occurs in consequence of weakness of the muscles of the lower portion of the abdomen. The fibers of these muscles are apt to separate, when a sudden muscular effort is made, thus permitting the intestine to protude. In some cases the truss has been dispensed with, and the difficulty removed, through the strengthening processes of the duplicated movement.

The proper movement for self-treatment is Number 51, half-stretch, half-wing, half-kick step-standing, trunk twisting. This movement is at first to be performed with one side only, the trunk twisting toward the relaxed side—that is, the side of which the foot is raised. After some progress is made, the twisting should be done in the opposite direction. The kneeling twisting, movement is especially helpful.

Chronic Backache

When the backache is caused by fatigue, those movements which involve the abdominal muscles are useful. This problem is often caused by laxity of muscles, allowing the visceral contents to gravitate. In this case movement numbers 43, 48, 56, 36, 30, and 31 are recommended.

21   Conclusion

The ethos of treating the whole person has hit an exposed nerve in this country which spends approximately $287 billion a year on medical care and, if we are to believe such experts as Franz J. Ingelfinger, former editor of *The New England Journal of Medicine*, spends so abundantly at the same time that 80 percent of patients are unaffected by treatment.

To some extent, clearly, people can influence their health by what they do and in many cases by what they think. This book, which views health as a condition reflecting interaction among a patient's background, environment, state of mind and the disease or injury, reflects not only a dissatisfaction with modern medicine and its dependence on drugs as a panacea for all our ills, but a deep desire to find and use alternative therapies.

It is to the fulfillment of this desire that Holistic Health is dedicated. A doctor's real duty is to teach people how to stay well. In order to be truly healthy and live well and long, we must exercise sensibly, eat frugally from a diet of natural foods, minimize stress, regenerate our physical and mental spirits and cultivate the laws of nature. The laws of nature cure and heal, doctors don't. All a doctor can do is offer advice on how to speed up the process of getting well. Remember he or she can't put new cells in the body, repair bones, or sew together torn ligaments.

Holistic healing, then, respects the body's ability to heal itself. The body can create the vital energy we all desire and seek. Diet, exercise and positive thinking are important, as is stress management and proper attention to the physical self, to the mind, and to the soul. In our country today, reckless and improper lifestyles impair and shorten tens of millions of lives. These are not the horrible starving diseases of the Third World such as rickets, scurvy, beri beri and pellagra; ours are the slower, more insidious killers that modern society has fostered: heart and circulatory disorders, many types of cancer and diabetes, stress, certain types of schizophrenia, autism and other mental afflictions. Many of these ills are created by government failures: decaying cities, acid rain, and unchecked chemical infiltration of our air. These are failures which our present health care custodians cannot control either. Which is perhaps why, in a poll conducted in 1980 by the National Opinion Research Center, only 52 percent of Americans felt a "great deal" of confidence in doctors. A recent survey conducted by the Institute for Complementary Medicine found the number of patients turning to alternative therapies growing at an annual rate of 15 percent.

Our new nationwide preoccupation—some say obsession—with health has led to a passion for jogging, physical fitness, pursuit of nutritionally whole foods, and concern about chemical pollution which seems to suggest that once again the general population and not the medical and scientific bureacracy has recognized the value of a new plan for national health.

We who are holistic health proponents believe that there is more evidence today than ever before of the mind-body link, and that in order to really measure health we must speak of both physical and psychological well-being. There are many social and emotional nutrients of which I have spoken in this book, among them are movements and recreation, meditation and affection, proteins, vitamins, herbs and organic nutrition. These are vital components of total health for us all.

Above all else, if we are to practice true holistic living, we must learn to live in harmony with ourselves—body and soul, each other, and nature as a whole. We are talking here about a way of life and not a prescription to be filled at a local pharmacy. Whatever ambitions you dream of fulfilling you must have health. And I believe the theories recounted in this book can save, prolong, or improve your life as they have mine.

FIGURES

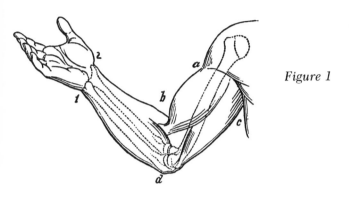

Figure 1

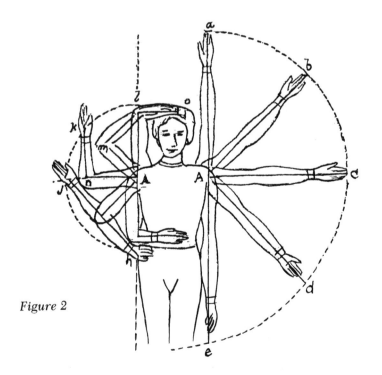

Figure 2

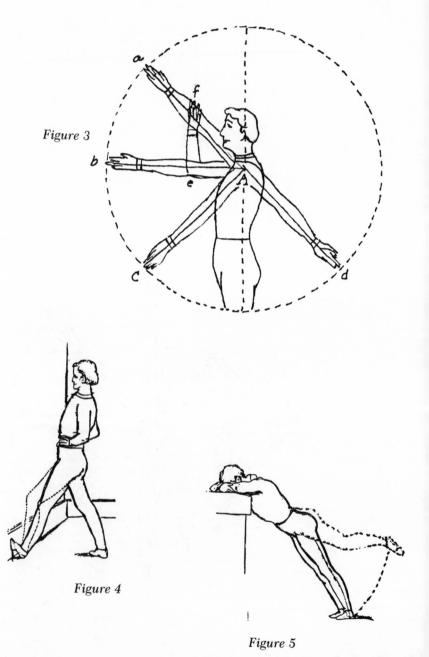

Figure 3

Figure 4

Figure 5

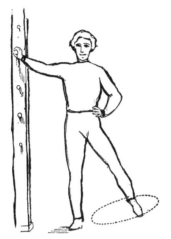

Figure 6

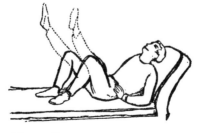

Figure 7

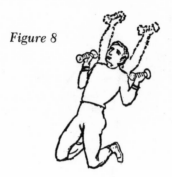

Figure 8

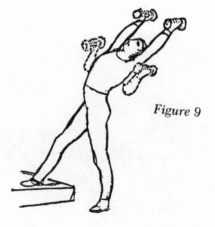

Figure 9

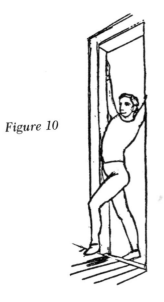

Figure 10

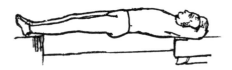

Figure 11

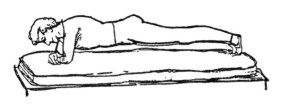

Figure 12

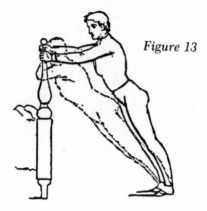

Figure 13

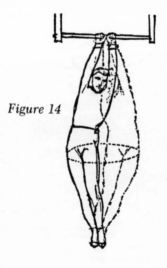

Figure 14

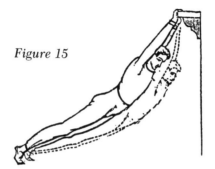

Figure 15

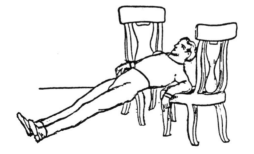

Figure 16

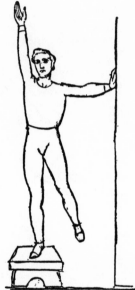

Figure 17

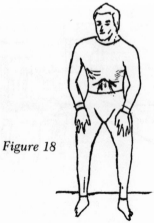

Figure 18

GLOSSARY

ARTHRITIS. Inflammation of a joint.

ASANA. Yoga postures.

ANTEVERSION. Forward tipping or tilting of an organ.

AMENORRHEA. Absence or abnormal stoppage of the menses.

ANEMIA. A condition in which the blood is deficient either in quantity or quality.

CHILBLAINS. A localized itching and painful erythema of fingers, toes or ears produced by cold, damp weather: a disease of the small blood vessels of the skin.

CORPOREAL. Having a body.

CEREBROSPINAL. Pertaining to the brain and the spinal cord.

DYSPEPSIA. Among other things, an impairment of the power or function of digestion.

EMPHYSEMA. Pertaining to the lungs, a swelling or inflation due to the presence of air in the interstices of the connective tissues, and others.

FAUCES. Passage from the mouth to the pharynx.

FASCIA. A sheet of fibrous tissue which covers the body under the skin and invests the muscles and certain organs.

FEBRILE. Pertaining to a fever.

HEMIPLEGIA. Paralysis on one side of the body.

HERNIA. A protrusion of a loop of an organ or tissue through an abnormal opening.

INNERVATION. The distribution or supply of nerves to a part.

KELP. A sea weed.

MORPHOLOGICAL. A branch of biology which treats form and structure.

METAMORPHOSIS. A passing from one form or shape to another.

NEURALGIA. Paroxysmal pain which extends along the course of the nerves.

PERINEUM. The region of the body between the genital organs and the rectum.

PROLAPSUS. A falling down or out.

RETROVERSION. Backward tipping or tilting of an organ.

SENSORIUM. The nervous system including the cerebrum.

SEMINAL DISEASE. This pertains to the seed or to the semen.

VITO-CHEMICAL. Pertaining to organic chemical.

YOGA. A Hindu system of mystical and physical philosophy that involves withdrawal from the physical world and meditation upon some object..

SELECTED BIBLIOGRAPHY

Duke, Marc. *Acupuncture*. New York: Pyramid House Books, 1972.

Dorland's *Medical Dictionary*. 23rd ed. Philadelphia: W.B. Saunders Co.

Duke, Robert E. *Hypnotherapy for Troubled Children*. New York: New Horizon Press & Irvington Publishers, Inc., 1983.

Dunne, Desmond. *Yoga*. New York: Wilfred Funk, 1953.

Frose, Brodel, Schlossberg. *Human Anatomy*. New York: Barnes & Noble, Inc.

Lee & Whincup. *Chinese Massage Therapy*. Boulder: Shambhala Publications Inc., 1983.

Ling, Peter H. Treatise on Gymnastics Without Apparatus. Sweden:

Powers, Melvin. *Hypnosis Revealed*. No. Hollywood: Wilshire Book Co.

Rothstein, H. *Gymnastics in Sweden*.

———— The *Gymnastic System of Ling*.

Taylor, M.D., George. *The Movement Cure*. New York: Fowler & Wells Publishers.

Index of Holistic Movements

INDEX